Plastic and Aesthetic Nursing

Third Edition

Scope and Standards of Practice

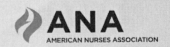

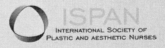

The International Society of Plastic and Aesthetic Nurses (ISPAN) and the American Nurses Association (ANA) are national professional associations. This joint ISPAN and ANA publication—*Plastic and Aesthetic Nursing: Scope and Standards of Practice, 3rd Edition*—reflects the position of the ISPAN regarding the specialty practice of plastic and aesthetic nursing and should be reviewed in conjunction with state board of nursing regulations. State law, rules, and regulations govern the practice of nursing, while *Plastic and Aesthetic Nursing: Scope and Standards of Practice, 3rd Edition* guides plastic and aesthetic registered nurses in the application of their professional skills and responsibilities.

About the International Society of Plastic and Aesthetic Nurses
The International Society of Plastic and Aesthetic Nurses (ISPAN) is committed to the enhancement of quality nursing care delivered to the patient undergoing plastic and reconstructive surgery and nonsurgical aesthetic procedures. ISPAN promotes high standards of plastic and aesthetic nursing practice and patient care through education, scientific inquiry, analysis and dissemination of information. For more information: https://ISPAN.org/

About the American Nurses Association
The American Nurses Association (ANA) is the only full-service professional organization representing the interests of the nation's 4 million registered nurses through its constituent/state nurses associations and its organizational affiliates. The ANA advances the nursing profession by fostering high standards of nursing practice, promoting the rights of nurses in the workplace, projecting a positive and realistic view of nursing, and by lobbying the Congress and regulatory agencies on health care issues affecting nurses and the public.

American Nurses Association
8515 Georgia Avenue, Suite 400
Silver Spring, MD 20910

ISBN   SAN: 851-3481
Print 978-1-947800-71-7
epdf 978-1-947800-72-4
epub 978-1-947800-73-1
mobi 978-1-947800-74-8

Contents

Contributors

International Society of Plastic and Aesthetic Nurses (ISPAN) Scope and Standards Task Force

Kathleen Soso, MSN, RN, CPSN-R, ISPAN-F, Chair

Sharon Ann Van Wicklin, PhD, RN, CNOR, CRNFA(E), CPSN-R, PLNC, FAAN, ISPAN-F

Dawn P. Sagrillo, MSN, AGNP-C, CANS, CPSN, ISPAN-F

ANA Staff

Carol J. Bickford, PhD, RN-BC, CPHIMS, FHIMSS, FAAN—Content editor

Erin E. Walpole, BA, PMP—Project editor

ANA Committee on Nursing Practice Standards

Nena M. Bonuel, PhD, RN, CCRN-K, APRN-BC

Patricia Bowe, DNP, MS, RN

Danette Culver, MSN, APRN, ACNS-BC, CCRN

Elizabeth O. Dietz, EdD, RN, CS-NP, Alternate

Kirk Koyama, MSN, RN, CNS, PHN, Co-Chair

Tonette McAndrew, MPA, RN

Stacy McNall, MSN, RN, IBCLC

Verna Sitzer, PhD, RN, CNS

Mona Pearl Treyball, PhD, RN, CNS, CCRN-K, FAAN

Jordan Wilson, BSN, RN, Alternate

About the International Society of Plastic and Aesthetic Nurses

The International Society of Plastic and Aesthetic Nurses (ISPAN) is committed to the enhancement of quality nursing care delivered to the client undergoing plastic and reconstructive surgery and nonsurgical aesthetic procedures. ISPAN promotes high standards of plastic and aesthetic nursing practice and client care through education, scientific inquiry, analysis, and dissemination of information.

About the American Nurses Association

The American Nurses Association (ANA) is the only full-service professional organization representing the interests of the nation's 4 million registered nurses through its constituent/state nurses' associations and its organizational affiliates. The ANA advances the nursing profession by fostering high standards of nursing practice, promoting the rights of nurses in the workplace, projecting a positive and realistic view of nursing, and by lobbying the Congress and regulatory agencies on health care issues affecting nurses and the public.

Scope of Plastic and Aesthetic Nursing Practice

Definition of Plastic and Aesthetic Nursing

Plastic and aesthetic nursing specializes in the protection, maintenance, safety, and optimization of health and human bodily restoration and repair before, during, and after plastic cosmetic and reconstructive surgical procedures or nonsurgical aesthetic procedures. This is accomplished through the nursing process (i.e., assessment, diagnosis, outcomes identification, planning, implementation, evaluation). The plastic and aesthetic registered nurse (RN) collaborates, consults, and serves as a liaison and advocate for individuals, families, groups, communities, and populations and bridges the role of the plastic and aesthetic RN with that of other professionals to promote optimal holistic client outcomes and improve the well-being of the client.

Foundation of Plastic and Aesthetic Nursing

The specialty of plastic and aesthetic nursing has long pioneered treatment strategies for human body and facial repair, reconstruction, and replacement in cases of congenital deformities or diseases, traumatic injuries, and removal of tissue due to cancer or disease. Minimally invasive, nonsurgical cosmetic or aesthetic procedures are an essential component of the specialty that are used both to improve overall appearance and to optimize the outcome of reconstructive surgical procedures. Additionally, these interventions may serve to rejuvenate and/or correct aesthetic concerns of the client and may also postpone effects of the aging process.

Plastic and aesthetic sites include the skin, breast, trunk, cranio-maxillofacial structures, musculoskeletal system, extremities, and external genitalia. Plastic and aesthetic interventions focus on the care of complex wounds, replants, grafts, flaps, free tissue transfers, use of implantable materials, and the healing process and response. Plastic and aesthetic interventions encompass clients of all ages, from the neonate to the oldest adult healthcare client.

As a result of their specialized education and training, plastic and aesthetic RNs are aware of the health risks and potential complications associated with plastic and aesthetic procedures. As members of the interprofessional healthcare team, plastic and aesthetic RNs complement the specialty by maintaining a focus on healthcare client safety, health maintenance, optimal outcomes, and client satisfaction. Increasing societal awareness of plastic and aesthetic procedures requires the leadership and expertise of plastic and aesthetic RNs to clarify misconceptions, provide education, and execute procedures with a high degree of skill, as well as to protect individuals, families, groups, communities, and populations from unnecessary health and safety risks.

Plastic and aesthetic nursing practice and standards reflect the nursing process, the nursing standards of the American Nurses Association (ANA, 2015a), the guidelines (2019) and standards (2015) of the Association of periOperative Registered Nurses (AORN), and the standards of the American Society of PeriAnesthesia Nurses (2019-2020).

Plastic and aesthetic nursing requires specialized knowledge and skills for both the reconstructive and aesthetic aspects of surgical interventions during the client's initial consultation, and during the preoperative, intraoperative, and postoperative stages of the surgical or aesthetic procedure. Another level of specialized knowledge and skills is required of aesthetic RNs who perform and/or assist with aesthetic procedures. Through the implementation and maintenance of specialized plastic and aesthetic nursing standards of practice, individuals seeking or undergoing plastic surgery interventions and/or aesthetic treatments and procedures can be provided with education, knowledge, and nursing care designed to promote optimal client safety and outcomes.

Growth of Plastic and Aesthetic Nursing Practice

Plastic and aesthetic nursing opportunities continue to expand as the demand for plastic surgical and nonsurgical aesthetic treatments and procedures grows. As shown in Figure 1, the number of annual cosmetic, reconstructive, and nonsurgical aesthetic procedures has grown steadily since 2005. According to the American Society of Plastic Surgeons (ASPS; 2019), more than 39.8 million plastic and aesthetic treatments and procedures were performed in 2018 (see Table 1), compared to 24.0 million in 2005, representing a 65.8% increase. The need for nursing knowledge related to plastic and aesthetic procedures, safety, quality, and ethical issues will continue to increase as plastic surgical and nonsurgical aesthetic treatments and procedures become more prevalent in a wide range of environments.

According to the ASPS (2018) survey of their board-certified plastic surgeons, the top three requested procedures in plastic surgery continue to be breast augmentation, abdominoplasty, and liposuction. Neuromodulators (botulinum toxin type A) will continue to be the most commonly requested minimally invasive procedure, followed by dermal fillers, chemical peels, laser hair removal, dermabrasion, non-invasive fat reduction, and non-surgical skin tightening. Emerging industry and related consumer trends in the field of aesthetic and plastic surgery will include advancements in skin tightening, scar management, and fat grafting.

With an increase in the number of clients seeking cosmetic surgical enhancement abroad, the American Society for Aesthetic Plastic Surgery (2019) has established guidelines for patients seeking cosmetic procedures that include:

- verifying the physician has specific training in cosmetic surgery through an accredited plastic surgery residency program or fellowship,
- obtaining clarity about who will be providing postoperative care and who is financially responsible for secondary or revisional procedures, and
- understanding what liability coverage the physician holds and what the local laws are relative to medical malpractice.

Plastic and aesthetic nurses may also participate in the care of clients who have experienced adverse outcomes from receiving aesthetic or reconstructive surgery abroad. Cosmetic surgery performed in developing countries carries significant risks for complications that can present significant burdens on the health system (Ross, Moscoso, Bayer, Rosselli-Risal, & Orgill, 2018). The ASPS (2012) has established the following cautionary statements for those individuals seeking medical tourism:

- Vacation-related activities may compromise patients' health.
- Cosmetic surgery is real surgery.
- Travel combined with surgery significantly increases risk of complications.
- Quality critical care facilities are not always available.
- Follow-up care and monitoring may be limited.
- Bargain surgery can be costly.
- Surgeon and facility qualifications may not be verifiable.
- Devices and products used may not meet U.S. standards.

As patient advocates and educators, plastic and aesthetic nurses have a responsibility to caution those considering aesthetic or reconstructive surgery abroad.

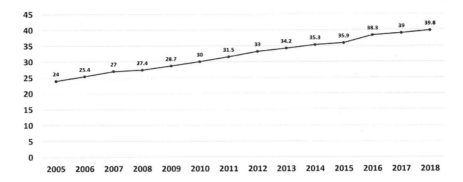

FIGURE 1.   Plastic Surgical and Aesthetic Procedures
in Millions (2005–2018).

Source: American Society of Plastic Surgeons. Plastic Surgery Statistics. https://
www.plasticsurgery.org/news/plastic-surgery-statistics.

TABLE 1.   Plastic Surgical and Aesthetic Procedures in
Millions by Type (2005–2018).

Year	Cosmetic	Reconstructive	Aesthetic (Nonsurgical)	Total	% Increase
2005	10.2	5.4	8.4	24.0	
2006	11.0	5.3	9.1	25.4	5.8
2007	11.8	5.2	10.0	27.0	6.3
2008	12.1	4.9	10.4	27.4	1.5
2009	12.5	5.2	11.0	28.7	4.7
2010	13.1	5.3	11.6	30.0	4.5
2011	13.8	5.5	12.2	31.5	5.0
2012	14.6	5.6	13.0	33.2	5.4
2013	15.1	5.7	13.4	34.2	3.0
2014	15.6	5.8	13.9	35.3	3.2
2015	15.9	5.8	14.2	35.9	1.7
2016	17.1	5.8	15.4	38.3	6.7
2017	17.5	5.8	15.7	39.0	1.8
2018	18.1	5.8	15.9	39.8	2.0

Source: American Society of Plastic Surgeons. Plastic Surgery Statistics.
https://www.plasticsurgery.org/news/plastic-surgery-statistics.

Development of Plastic and Aesthetic Nursing Practice

In response to the unique needs of plastic surgery healthcare clients and the specialized nursing interventions necessary for safe and effective practice, 100 surgical RNs convened in 1975 to establish the nonprofit organization called the American Society of Plastic and Reconstructive Surgical Nurses (ASPRSN). In 2001 ASPRSN simplified its name to the American Society of Plastic Surgical Nurses (ASPSN). In 2017, in an effort to emphasize the strong presence of members who practice in the aesthetic realm and to recognize members who practice outside of the United States, ASPSN changed its name to the International Society of Plastic and Aesthetic Nurses (ISPAN). The mission and philosophy of the ASPRSN were founded on principles aimed at improving the quality of nursing care for the healthcare client undergoing plastic or reconstructive surgery; that mission has evolved to include nursing care of health care clients undergoing nonsurgical aesthetic procedures as well.

The organization continues its commitment to promoting high standards of nursing care and practice through shared knowledge, scientific inquiry, and continuing education, while supporting and encouraging collaborative interaction with leaders in clinical practice, administration, research, and academics. The chronology of the development of plastic and aesthetic nursing is summarized in Table 2.

Currently, the ISPAN has more than 1,000 active members working in various nursing environments that include surgery centers, home care, nursing research, outpatient care, hospitals, universities, private practice, nonsurgical aesthetics centers, and others. Members of ISPAN are academically prepared at a wide range of educational levels, including associate, baccalaureate, master's, and doctoral degrees. Members hold numerous roles, such as advanced practice RN, RN first assistant, and RN educator. ISPAN serves its members through an international structure of chapters in the United States and Canada.

The ISPAN is truly an international organization with participation from plastic and aesthetic RNs located throughout the world. The society's professional publication, *Plastic Surgical Nursing*, features articles written by RNs practicing internationally. Additionally, the publisher offers authors the ability to develop their articles in their primary language and then have the work translated into English for dissemination throughout the plastic and aesthetic nursing world (ISPAN, 2019). The position statements developed by the Clinical Practice Committee for the ISPAN organization highlight the variations in scopes of practice for RNs from state to state and country to country and mandate that plastic and aesthetic RNs adhere to local, state, and federal regulations pertaining to scope of practice (ISPAN, 2018). This scope and standards document has been created to provide guidance for all RNs caring for plastic and aesthetic healthcare clients, regardless of the country in which this care is provided.

TABLE 2. Plastic and Aesthetic Nursing: A Chronology

Year	Event
1975	The American Society of Plastic and Reconstructive Surgical Nurses (ASPRSN) holds its first national meeting in Toronto, Canada.
	Sherill Lee Schultz is the first president and founder.
1976	Thirteen local chapters of ASPRSN are established in the United States and Canada.
1980	ASPRSN created *Plastic Surgical Nursing*.
	ASPRSN became the 22nd member of the National Federation for Specialty Nursing Organizations.
1984	The plastic surgical nursing bibliography was completed.
1989	The first edition of the *Core Curriculum for Plastic and Reconstructive Surgical Nursing* was published.
	The Plastic Surgical Nursing Certification Board (PSNCB) was established.
1991	The first plastic surgical nursing certification examination (CPSN) was administered.
1995	ASPRSN established a Research Committee to assist ASPRSN nurses with research funds and priorities unique to plastic surgical nursing practice.
1996	The second edition of the *Core Curriculum for Plastic and Reconstructive Surgical Nursing* was published.
1998	ASPRSN created a website: www.aspsn.org
2001	ASPRSN simplified its name to the American Society of Plastic Surgical Nurses (ASPSN).
2004	The specialty was recognized by the American Nurses Association (ANA) and the collaborative ASPSN-ANA specialty standards document, *Plastic Surgery Nursing: Scope and Standards of Practice* was drafted.
2005	*Plastic Surgery Nursing: Scope and Standards of Practice* was published by Nursesbooks.org.
2007	The third edition of the *Core Curriculum for Plastic and Reconstructive Surgical Nursing* was published.
2010	A task force was initiated to develop an aesthetic nursing certification.
	A workgroup was convened to review and revise *Plastic Surgery Nursing: Scope and Standards of Practice*.
2011	The second edition of *Plastic Surgery Nursing: Scope and Standards of Practice* was published by Nursesbooks.org.
2013	The Certified Aesthetic Nurse Specialist (CANS) designation and exam were created and administered.
2014	The fourth edition of the *Core Curriculum for Plastic and Reconstructive Surgical Nursing* was published.
2016	A new logo was selected to reflect the changing landscape of plastic surgical nursing.
2017	A new name (International Society of Plastic and Aesthetic Nurses [ISPAN]) was adopted to reflect inclusion of aesthetic practitioners and members of international chapters (www.ispan.org).
	A new mission, vision, and society values were developed to emphasize that the Society is the definitive voice of plastic surgical nursing.
2018	A workgroup was convened to review and revise *Plastic Surgery Nursing: Scope and Standards of Practice*.
	New nomenclature (Plastic and Aesthetic Nursing) was developed to reflect the more inclusive name, mission, and vision of the ISPAN.

Through the development of specialized knowledge, the plastic and aesthetic RN can effectively respond to and communicate with an interdisciplinary team assigned to care for any plastic or aesthetic healthcare client. As the field of plastic surgery evolves and interacts with other specialties, the climate for plastic and aesthetic nursing requires ongoing review of related trends, products, and procedures. Due to the continued steady growth in plastic and aesthetic procedures, there will be an ongoing need for skilled and knowledgeable RNs within the highly challenging yet rewarding area of plastic and aesthetic nursing.

Plastic and Aesthetic Nurses and Healthcare Clients

The plastic and aesthetic RN provides competent and ethical nursing care to improve clients' experiences and outcomes. One goal of plastic and aesthetic nursing is to provide a foundation of practice based on client safety. This is accomplished through strong regulations, as well as effective education and awareness programs for healthcare clients, families, groups, communities, and populations seeking or requiring plastic and aesthetic interventions. Because of the physical and psychological complexities involved in caring for individuals undergoing cosmetic, reconstructive, and nonsurgical aesthetic procedures, plastic and aesthetic RNs must integrate a holistic approach into the plan of care for the healthcare client. To determine and implement the plan of care, and to help ensure optimal outcomes, the plastic and aesthetic RN encourages and facilitates consultations, communication, and collaboration with other healthcare team members.

Plastic and aesthetic RNs promote and improve quality of care before, during, and after plastic and aesthetic procedures and treatments to help ensure effective health maintenance, safety, and restoration. Plastic and aesthetic RNs determine the specific nursing interventions necessary for each individual undergoing a plastic or aesthetic procedure or treatment, in accordance with the nursing process. The plastic and aesthetic nursing specialty continues to develop and strengthen its knowledge base for providing evidence-based practice by researching and incorporating evidence and client input into plastic and aesthetic procedures, treatments, and client care.

The plastic and aesthetic RN interacts with and cares for healthcare clients who require or desire plastic surgery or nonsurgical aesthetic treatments for enhancement or restoration purposes. The plastic and aesthetic RN also interacts with and educates healthcare clients, families, and populations regarding plastic and aesthetic procedures, treatments, and other related issues. The plastic and aesthetic RN has the specialized knowledge and skills necessary to meet the needs of the healthcare client population.

The plastic and aesthetic RN provides care in a variety of settings and with a variety of age groups and populations, including pediatric clients and older adults, individuals undergoing all types of surgery, and those who have sustained traumatic injuries. Plastic and aesthetic RNs provide nursing care and education to help healthcare clients obtain a thorough understanding of procedures, achieve realistic personal expectations, and participate in mutual goal setting.

The care of pediatric clients undergoing plastic and aesthetic procedures is extremely complex. The plastic and aesthetic RN cares not only for the client, but also for the client's parent/guardian/caregiver (Gart, 2014). Pediatric clients typically pursue plastic and aesthetic care for the treatment of congenital disorders, including cleft lip and palate, burns, congenital hand and craniofacial deformities, and removal of congenital lesions of the skin; the management of these disorders requires expertise from a multidisciplinary, interprofessional team (Gart, 2014; Heike et al., 2010; LoGiudice & Gosain, 2004; Sullivan & Adkinson, 2016; Svientek & Levine, 2015). Additionally, the pediatric client may require multiple interventions and revisions of prior procedures as the client continues to develop and mature. It is the responsibility of the plastic and aesthetic RN to coordinate care that ensures the administration of appropriate treatments and interventions at the appropriate time in the client's development (Gart, 2014).

The plastic and aesthetic RN provides care to clients as they advance throughout the lifespan; many clients seek care for concerns and changes related to the effects of aging (Brennan, 2018). The assessment of clients seeking treatment to minimize or reverse the physiological effects of aging must also include a thorough review of any medical conditions/comorbidities and medication reconciliation; any treatments or interventions recommended by the plastic and aesthetic RN must take these complicating factors into consideration (Brennan, 2018). Certain medical conditions, such as autoimmune disorders, and over the counter or prescribed medications that have anticoagulation properties, may limit or delay the treatment options available to these clients (Brennan, 2018). The plastic and aesthetic RN is also obligated to communicate honestly and compassionately when working to manage any unrealistic expectations held by the older adult client. The older adult client seeking plastic and aesthetic nursing care requires comprehensive clinical management and psychological support.

Plastic and aesthetic RNs help healthcare clients deal with perceived or altered body image, expected surgical outcomes, personal fears, and individual learning needs associated with the desired surgical or nonsurgical intervention. The success of a plastic and/or aesthetic procedure cannot be evaluated without consideration of the client's perception of the outcomes; improvement of a client's psychological functioning through the alteration of that client's body image is a primary goal of plastic and aesthetic procedures (Rankin & Mayers, 2008). Healthcare clients undergoing plastic and aesthetic procedures or treatments may encounter psychological, emotional, and physical imbalances during the postoperative phase. Managing the psychological discord associated with physical alterations requires specialized nursing knowledge and education.

In the United States, beauty is defined by the media through television, music, magazines, and the Internet (Hass, Champion, & Secor, 2008). The majority of these sources send messages about how to improve one's appearance by dieting, exercising or undergoing cosmetic procedures (Hass et al., 2008). Because only a small portion of individuals meet this standard, individuals are driven to pursue unrealistic goals (Haas et al., 2008). As the demand for cosmetic surgical and nonsurgical procedures increases, it is important for plastic and aesthetic RNs to recognize the motive behind the client's decision to undergo these procedures.

In a synthesis of the literature to understand the reasons that people elect to undergo cosmetic surgery, Haas et al. (2008), found that the most common motivating factors included body dysmorphic disorder, body image, self-esteem, teasing, and media influence. People with body dysmorphic disorder perceive themselves as ugly and become obsessed with a particular perceived defect that is very minor and may even be unnoticeable to others. These individuals may desire cosmetic procedures to improve their appearance and may return repeatedly for multiple procedures. Changing one's body image may also be a significant motivator for undergoing cosmetic procedures. Social acceptance, and the anticipation of receiving positive feedback from friends and acquaintances following a cosmetic procedure can improve self-esteem and motivate individuals to undergo cosmetic procedures. People with a history of being teased about their appearance may also undergo cosmetic procedures in an effort to gain acceptance or approval from their peers. The media portrays the ideal woman as being slim and muscular with large breasts. Because this figure occurs in only a small percentage of women, they may seek cosmetic surgery in hopes of achieving a similar standard of beauty, or in hopes of looking like a particular celebrity. Plastic and aesthetic RNs should be cognizant of the need for obtaining a thorough history and physical examination and ensuring sufficient time spent in consultation with the client to make the best decision about whether the client is an appropriate candidate for the elective cosmetic procedure.

Although body piercing has been popular for many centuries and with many cultures, over the past few decades, the practice of ear gauging, a traditional tribal practice, has become popular in western society, especially among adolescents (Henderson & Malata, 2010; Pek, Goh, & Pek, 2017; Snell & Caplash, 2013). Those who have undergone ear gauging may find themselves being discriminated against in various facets of life (Snell & Caplash, 2013). Career choices, parental pressure, and increasing age have led to individuals regretting their ear lobe expansion and seeking to have their ears restored to normal

(Henderson & Malata, 2010; Pek, Goh, & Pek, 2017; Snell & Caplash, 2013). Plastic and aesthetic RNs should be aware that this procedure has an inherent risk of hypertrophic scars or keloids (Pek et al., 2017). Obtaining photographs from the client to show what their ears looked like before the ear gauging process can be helpful in guiding the surgeon in restoring the appearance of the lobe (Henderson & Malata, 2010).

Approximately one third of adults in the United States have at least one tattoo, and of those persons with tattoos, 69% have more than one (Shannon-Missal, 2018). Tattoos are most common among younger individuals, with almost 50% of millennials having at least one tattoo (Shannon-Missal, 2018). Tattooing is currently accepted as a fashionable mode of self-expression or sharing life experiences and cherished memories that is widely practiced by individuals from diverse socioeconomic and ethnic backgrounds (Farley, Van Hoover, & Rademeyer, 2019). Despite increasing mainstream acceptance of this art form, people with tattoos may experience stigma, stereotyping, and discrimination in their personal and professional lives (Farley et al., 2019). Tattoos have also been used as an indication of group membership (e.g., military) as well as a mark of ownership or subservience (e.g., identification numbers on concentration camp victims, women trapped in sex trafficking; Sidner, 2017). For victims who were tattooed without consent, tattoo removal or revision can provide a way to heal (Survivor's Ink, 2017).

Approximately 50% of people with a tattoo regret having the tattoo, and more than 20% desire removal (Islam et al., 2016). Before the individual undergoes tattoo removal, plastic and aesthetic nurses should explore the client's goals and establish realistic expectations (Ho & Goh, 2015). The client should be educated about potential complications, side effects, and expected outcomes.

The scope of practice of the plastic and aesthetic RN includes the care of clients who have sustained burn injuries. The care of a burn client requires a comprehensive and multidisciplinary approach (Svientek & Levine, 2015). Stabilization and fluid resuscitation are the initial goals of the plastic and aesthetic RN. Then promotion of wound healing, psychological and emotional support, and prevention of wound contractures become the primary focus of the plastic and aesthetic RN; as the burn injury heals, the plastic and aesthetic RN coordinates care to include physical therapy to promote functionality and emotional support to facilitate coping (Svientek & Levine, 2015).

Treatments to address the obesity epidemic include bariatric surgeries where successful client outcomes include massive weight loss over an abbreviated period of time (Wakefield, Rubin, & Gusenoff, 2014). The plastic and aesthetic RN's scope of practice includes caring for clients who require removal of excess loose skin and body contouring procedures. A thorough assessment must be conducted to determine the client's weight stability; surgical interventions to contour the body should ideally be scheduled after the client has maintained the massive weight loss and current weight for approximately 1 year (Wakefield et al., 2014). The plastic and aesthetic RN should collaborate and communicate with the client's bariatric surgeon, nutritionist, and primary care providers to ensure appropriate nutritional and weight management throughout the perioperative process. Additionally, the plastic and aesthetic RN must assess the client's self-image to identify potential body dysmorphia or unrealistic expectations that should be addressed preoperatively; this may necessitate the requirement of preoperative clearance from a mental health professional (Wakefield et al., 2014). Bariatric patients who have sustained massive weight loss may require multiple surgical procedures to remove loose or hanging skin, and the plastic and aesthetic RN plays a pivotal role in the coordination of these procedures.

Plastic and aesthetic RNs coordinate the care of clients undergoing reconstruction after excision of malignancies; these malignancies include breast cancers, skin cancers, and carcinomas (Garcia-Vilarino et al., 2018; Rudolph & Miller, 2000; Steffen, Johnson, Levine, Mayer, & Avis, 2017). The goals of care for these clients include management of the physiological threat of disease and improvement of quality of life through the restoration of physical appearance (Steffen et al., 2017). In addition to the administering perioperative nursing care, the plastic and aesthetic RN must also collaborate within the interdisciplinary and multispecialty team to ensure that surgical interventions are appropriately scheduled with consideration given to oncological treatments such as radiation and chemotherapy (Garcia-Vilarino et al., 2018).

An expanding client population that the plastic and aesthetic RN may encounter is the transgender client population seeking gender confirming surgeries. This is a field that is developing both within the United States and internationally (Berli et al., 2017). It requires coordination of care across many disciplines, including plastic surgery, endocrinology, primary care, psychology, urology, and gynecology. The plastic and aesthetic RN should coordinate care to ensure ideal client outcomes from not only a physiological perspective, but also from a psychological and emotional aspect as well.

Plastic and aesthetic RNs should adhere to regulatory standards, professional guidelines, and evidence-based practices for pain management when caring for clients undergoing surgical or nonsurgical procedures. Preoperative pain management strategies may include implementing screening to identify high-risk clients and educating clients about postprocedural pain expectations and management (Glass, Hardy, Meeks, & Carroll, 2015). Intraoperative pain management strategies may include using regional blocks to reduce postoperative pain and toxicity risks associated with local anesthetics, buffering local anesthetics, administering anxiolytics, and administering nonsteroidal anti-inflammatory drugs (NSAIDs) to reduce pain and opioid requirements during the first 24 hours (Glass et al., 2015). Postoperative strategies for pain management may include administering NSAIDs for pain control to reduce opioid requirements and using opioids as second line therapy (Glass et al., 2015).

Educational Preparation for Plastic and Aesthetic Nursing Roles

Prior to entering the specialty, plastic and aesthetic RNs are prepared at the associate, baccalaureate, master's, doctoral, or advanced practice registered nurse level. Plastic and aesthetic nursing knowledge and skills require a strong foundation in preoperative, intraoperative, and postoperative standards, guidelines, and practices; wound healing and wound care; safety and quality; anatomy and physiology; bioethics; and psychology. Broad experience in surgical duties, sterile technique, and perianesthesia care enhances the RN's ability to build on the skill sets required for a successful specialty practice.

Because there are no formal academic plastic or aesthetic nursing educational programs, plastic and aesthetic RNs often leverage the AORN and American Society of PeriAnesthesia Nurses (ASPAN) educational curriculum for perioperative and perianesthesia RNs.

The plastic and aesthetic RN learns about plastic surgery and aesthetic fundamentals from professional courses offered by ISPAN; core curriculum materials, mentoring, and educational seminars; workshops and hands-on training pertaining to plastic surgery and aesthetic procedures; and nursing care. Obtaining education and experience with plastic and aesthetic procedures and client outcomes will increase knowledge and help the RN attain the skills necessary to provide optimal care for the plastic and aesthetic healthcare client. Due to the complexities of the specialty, plastic and aesthetic RNs should obtain a minimum of two years of plastic and/or aesthetic nursing experience before seeking specialty certification. Nurses entering the specialty should also develop an understanding of psychological and psychosocial factors related to healthcare clients undergoing plastic and aesthetic procedures.

The Plastic Surgical Nursing Certification Board (PSNCB) offers two certifications for plastic and aesthetic RNs:

- Certified Plastic Surgery Nurse (CPSN)
- Certified Aesthetic Nurse Specialist (CANS)

Eligibility to sit for the certification exams includes current licensure as an RN in the United States or Canada, a minimum of 2 years and 1,000 hours of plastic or aesthetic experience, and current employment with a board-certified plastic/aesthetic surgeon, ophthalmologist, dermatologist, or facial plastic surgeon.

Minimum Requirements for the CPSN

- Licensure as an RN within the designated state of practice
- Education
  - Minimum requirement: Associate Degree in Nursing from an accredited college or university
  - Preferred: Bachelor of Science in Nursing from an accredited college or university
- Advanced knowledge in anatomy and physiology specific to all age groups
- Advanced knowledge in treatment of clients with
  - wounds, including complex wounds
  - burns
  - traumatic injury
  - cancer-related disfigurements
  - scars
  - body image concerns
- Knowledge of health assessment and nutrition
- Knowledge of perioperative principles and aseptic technique
- Knowledge and ongoing education related to current plastic surgery trends, treatments and procedures, and related issues
- Certification as CPSN (see psncb.org)

Minimum Requirements for the CANS

- Licensure as an RN within the designated state of practice
- Education
  - Minimum requirement: Associate Degree in Nursing from an accredited college or university
  - Preferred: Bachelor of Science in Nursing from an accredited college or university

- Work in collaboration or in a practice with a physician who is Board Certified in Plastic or Aesthetic Surgery, Ophthalmology, Oculoplastics, Dermatology, Facial Plastic Surgery, or Otorhinolaryngology (ENT)

- Advanced knowledge in anatomy and physiology specific to all age groups

- Knowledge of perioperative principles and aseptic technique

- Knowledge and ongoing education related to current aesthetic trends, treatments and procedures, products, and technologies

- Knowledge of specific state nursing scope of practice related to aesthetic procedures performed

- Certification as CANS (see psnccb.org)

Roles of Plastic and Aesthetic Registered Nurses

State laws, rules, and regulations govern the practice of nursing, while *Nursing: Scope and Standards of Practice, Third Edition* (ANA, 2015a), *Nursing's Social Policy Statement: The Essence of the Profession* (ANA, 2010), and *Code of Ethics for Nurses with Interpretive Statements* (ANA, 2015b) provide the foundation for all RNs and their professional practice. The roles of the plastic and aesthetic RN further derive from the specialty's scope of practice statement and specific standards of care, recommended educational guidelines, and practice environments. Although plastic and aesthetic RNs assume many different roles, and perform many tasks independently, they are also responsible for adhering to the regulations set forth by their state boards of nursing and the policies and procedures dictated by their healthcare organizations. It is essential for all RNs to practice within their RN scope of practice. Plastic and aesthetic RNs can use the RN Scope of Practice Decision Tree (see Figure 2) to help determine if a particular task is within their scope of practice.

One of the goals of plastic and aesthetic nursing is to educate RNs and nursing students about plastic surgical and nonsurgical aesthetic issues, procedures, and current trends. Communication and interaction with nursing students and RNs from other nursing specialties about plastic surgery and aesthetic nursing will provide a broader understanding of the specialty among RNs and a greater knowledge base for nursing collaboration.

Plastic and aesthetic RNs are also knowledgeable about policies, procedures, contracts, and regulations, including those for compliance with the Health Insurance Portability and Accountability Act (HIPAA) in plastic and aesthetic settings. Plastic and aesthetic RNs know and comply with the requirements for federal, state, and local regulations, as well as insurance and accreditation

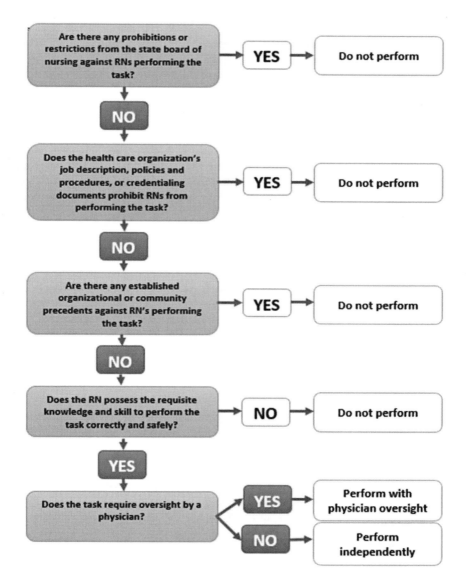

FIGURE 2.   RN Scope of Practice Decision Tree

Source: ISPAN RN Scope of Practice Decision Tree (2018). Reprinted with permission from ISPAN. Copyright © 2018. ISPAN, 500 Cummings Center, Suite 4400, Beverly, MA 01915. All rights reserved.

agency standards for plastic and aesthetic practice, regardless of the type of practice setting. Regulatory requirements pertinent to plastic and aesthetic RNs working in any environment may originate from the Centers for Medicare and Medicaid Services (CMS); Occupational Safety and Health Administration (OSHA); and the U.S. Food and Drug Administration (FDA).

General Nursing Role

RNs beginning clinical practice in their first year of licensure are encouraged to gain knowledge and develop skills associated with basic medical and surgical principles in preparation for later specialization in plastic or aesthetic nursing. RNs who enter the plastic and aesthetic specialty must have a well-rounded base of knowledge about a wide variety of healthcare client populations. Duties and skills required for RNs practicing in this specialty are as diverse as the specialty itself. The RN may be accountable for a variety of responsibilities in a variety of settings. The RN may provide hands-on client care relating to perioperative services, wound management, client assessment, and nonsurgical aesthetic treatments. Care may also be provided in the capacity of counseling, procedure coordination, and phone triage. A plastic and aesthetic RN may also be employed as a consultant or sales representative for treatments or products pertinent to the plastic and aesthetic industry. The scope of knowledge and skills required for plastic and aesthetic nursing varies with the area of practice interest, previous nursing experience, and level of educational preparation. The general plastic and aesthetic RN will progress into a more proficient role with experience, training, mentoring, and additional education.

Plastic and Aesthetic Advanced Practice Roles

Advanced practice plastic and aesthetic nursing roles are increasing in response to societal needs. Nurse practitioner (NP) and clinical nurse specialist (CNS) are two of the roles included in the term *advanced practice*. Advanced practice registered nurses (APRNs) play a significant role in meeting the needs of the plastic surgery and aesthetic healthcare client.

Advanced practice registered nurses working in plastic surgery and aesthetics are valuable in practice because of their ability to use independent judgment in clinical decision-making and to provide comprehensive, skilled, and high-quality advanced nursing care across the continuum. An APRN has the educational preparation and training to provide comprehensive health assessments, differential diagnoses, and treatments for healthcare clients receiving plastic surgical or aesthetic procedures.

The APRN is an advocate for health maintenance, health promotion, and wellness. Plastic and aesthetic APRNs serve as a resource and consultant to other healthcare disciplines regarding the specialty. Legislation has made prescriptive authority and third-party reimbursement possible for the APRN. The APRN is instrumental in facilitating and conducting research and plays a key role in implementing evidence-based practice and continuity of care for the plastic and aesthetic healthcare client. Duties and skills required for APRNs practicing in this role include implementing all aspects of client care relating to perioperative services, wound management, nonsurgical aesthetic treatments, and client assessment of the plastic or aesthetic client. The aesthetic APRN may practice independently or collaboratively with a physician providing all types of nonsurgical aesthetic treatments.

A plastic and aesthetic APRN is prepared to

- practice collaboratively with the plastic surgeon and other team members in various perioperative settings to ensure the healthcare client achieves safe and effective surgical outcomes,
- provide direct patient care as it relates to plastic or aesthetic surgical and nonsurgical procedures,
- provide client and community education and resources pertaining to plastic and aesthetic topics and related issues, and
- participate in clinical research relating to plastic and aesthetic treatments, devices and products, and medications.

This level of knowledge and skill is demonstrated by the additional competencies required for the advanced practice plastic and aesthetic RN in the Standards of Plastic and Aesthetic Nursing Practice.

Plastic and Aesthetic Nurse Educator Role

Even though all RNs are educators in their role of caring for healthcare clients, a plastic and aesthetic RN educator should be educated at the master's-degree level or higher with a focus on plastic and aesthetic nursing education. Education at the graduate level prepares the RN educator to assume leadership roles within complex health, educational, and organizational systems. According to the American Association of Colleges of Nursing (2011), the essentials of master's education in nursing delineate the knowledge and skills acquired by RNs prepared at the graduate level. These essentials include:

- Background for practice from Sciences and Humanities
- Organizational and Systems Leadership
- Quality Improvement and Safety

- Translating and Integrating Scholarship into Practice
- Informatics and Healthcare Technologies
- Health Policy and Advocacy
- Interprofessional Collaboration for Improving Patient and Population Health Outcomes
- Clinical Prevention and Population Health for Improving Health
- Master's-Level Nursing Practice (pp. 4-5)

This level of knowledge and skill is demonstrated by the additional competencies required for the graduate-level prepared plastic and aesthetic RN in the Standards of Plastic and Aesthetic Nursing Practice.

Plastic and aesthetic RN educators promote educational clarity, practice based on professional standards of care, and increased knowledge and safety related to plastic and aesthetic procedures and outcomes. They interact with other plastic and aesthetic RNs, RNs from other specialties, healthcare providers, students, healthcare clients, and the community.

A plastic and aesthetic RN educator with a graduate or doctoral degree is prepared to:

- facilitate and develop focused education, curricula, and research in plastic and aesthetic nursing;
- be compliant with and supportive of state educational requirements to teach at community college or university institutions;
- conduct a needs assessment to help establish educational requirements in various practice environments and settings;
- function as an educator and liaison between the plastic surgeon or APRN and the healthcare client to help ensure continuity of care, health promotion, and health maintenance;
- provide a climate conducive to learning and endeavor to involve learners in an active learning process;
- collect and analyze data to evaluate the effectiveness and outcomes of various educational strategies, and, if necessary, provide a revised plan to address educational shortcomings and problems;
- function as a member of an interprofessional team, consultant, change agent, leader, and resource to nursing and healthcare disciplines both within and outside of the plastic and aesthetic specialty;

- generate research and disseminate findings into education and practice;
- develop instructions, guidelines, materials, and programs for RNs during nursing school rotations, distance learning experiences, and in various practices, environments, and settings related to plastic surgery and aesthetics; and
- provide education and resources for local and national communities on relevant plastic or aesthetic topics and related issues.

Certified Aesthetic Nurse Specialist Role

Because the demand for procedures to maintain beauty and a youthful appearance has increased steadily since 2005, the development of new and improved nonsurgical aesthetic and minimally invasive technologies and FDA-cleared or approved products, and procedures have also grown. This has led to the development of the aesthetic RN role. With the increasing demand for these procedures, the role of the aesthetic RN becomes more important.

The aesthetic RN has a scope of knowledge more specialized to nonsurgical aesthetic procedures and healthcare clients seeking these procedures than the general plastic surgery RN. The aesthetic RN has also undergone specialized education and training in anatomy and physiology, procedural techniques, interventions, products, technologies, and assessment techniques specific to aesthetic minimally invasive nonsurgical care. The aesthetic RN also participates in ongoing education and training relevant to this specialized role. The scope of practice for the aesthetic RN differs within each state, based on their state board of nursing regulations and position statements from professional nursing organizations specific to aesthetic nursing practice that may or may not be instituted.

The aesthetic RN must be focused on maintaining the highest standards of clinical care, safety, client outcomes, and ethics and must always consider the healthcare client's specific needs, requests, budget, lifestyle, and expectations. The aesthetic healthcare client may hear about new products or procedures through popular and social media. Consequently, as a professional, the aesthetic RN must guide and educate the client to select appropriate products, procedures, or technologies and be cognizant of when it is appropriate to make necessary referrals to the physician. As these procedures are out of pocket expenses for the individual, the aesthetic RN has an obligation to avoid any real or perceived conflicts of interest and to recommend and provide only those procedures or products that are appropriate for the individual client.

Practice Environments for the Plastic and Aesthetic Nurse

The plastic and aesthetic RN provides care for healthcare clients and their families or caretakers in a variety of settings and locations that include hospitals, outpatient ambulatory surgery centers, office-based surgery centers, private practice, and nonsurgical aesthetic centers.

Hospitals

The plastic surgery RN working in the hospital environment may care for plastic surgery clients in a variety of specialty departments or units. These include emergency departments, operating rooms, surgical units, burn centers, critical care units, oncology units, neonatal or pediatrics units, and others. Plastic surgery nursing within the hospital environment is multidimensional and includes skills, functions, roles, and responsibilities that evolve from the body of knowledge specific to plastic surgery nursing.

Outpatient Settings

The plastic surgery RN working in the outpatient setting (e.g., ambulatory surgery centers, private practice) may provide nursing care during the consultation, preoperative, intraoperative, postoperative, and follow-up stages of the plastic or aesthetic procedure. In addition to nursing responsibilities, the outpatient plastic or aesthetic RN may have administrative responsibilities such as staffing, billing, insurance verification and predetermination, and insurance filing, as well as budgetary duties including purchasing of medical supplies and equipment. The plastic or aesthetic RN working in an outpatient setting may have responsibilities that include assessing the individual healthcare client's needs, developing educational material, assisting physicians or APRNs, and conducting client and personnel education.

Nonsurgical Aesthetic Centers

A nonsurgical aesthetic center is a combined medical office and day spa that operates under the supervision of a medical director. Nonsurgical aesthetic centers tend to have a more clinical atmosphere than day spas and typically offer a wide range of services and treatments, which include aesthetic injectables (neurotoxins and dermal fillers); minimally invasive thread lifting, lasers and light-based treatments; radiofrequency, cryolypolysis, other body contouring treatments; chemical peels and other clinical skin care services (e.g., microdermabrasion, microneedling, platelet-rich plasma therapy, sclerotherapy). Most nonsurgical aesthetic centers also provide comprehensive skin care education and offer medical grade skin care products.

The RN in the role of aesthetic nurse in these settings incorporates educational preparation, ongoing hands-on training, conferences, and industry-supported education in learning about new technologies and FDA-cleared or approved products relating to the procedures provided.

The aesthetic RN practices with the overseeing physician before practicing independently and is also individually accountable for her or his practice. The aesthetic RN must maintain an active, collaborative, interdependent relationship with the medical director of the nonsurgical aesthetics center. The aesthetic RN should utilize protocols that are developed collaboratively with the medical doctor to guide practice. The aesthetic RN should provide specific and accurate documentation of procedures and post-procedure follow-up. To help assure competency of the RN, the overseeing physician should perform and document periodic supervision and evaluation of the RN's performance. The aesthetic RN should utilize client feedback and the best available evidence to guide treatment options. The aesthetic RN should not have any conflicts of interest and should provide potential clients with truthful and accurate information.

Plastic and Aesthetic Nursing Research and Evidence-Based Practice

Evidence-based practice (EBP) is a scholarly and systematic problem-solving paradigm that results in the delivery of high-quality health care. To make the best clinical decisions using EBP, research findings are blended with internal evidence—including practice-generated data, clinical expertise, and healthcare client values and input—to achieve the best outcomes for individuals, groups, populations, and healthcare systems. Nursing research and EBP contribute to the body of knowledge and enhance healthcare client outcomes.

Plastic and aesthetic RNs should be aware of the evidence relative to positive and negative outcomes relative to the procedures performed in their practice. Results from studies conducted over 40 years have indicated that the majority of clients undergoing cosmetic surgery have positive outcomes and are satisfied with the results of their procedure (Edgerton, Jacobsen, & Meyer, 1960; Glatt, Sarwer, O'Hara, et al., 1999). The results of these studies have shown that cosmetic surgery clients experience an improvement in feelings of self-worth and self-esteem, a reduction in feelings of distress and shyness, and an improvement in overall quality of life. Likewise, Wang et al. (2016) found there was an improvement in the client's quality of life and self-esteem after aesthetic medical procedures.

Sarwer, Wadden, Pertschuk, and Whitaker (1998) suggested that the type of procedure and amount of surgical change are important predictors of client satisfaction. Procedures involving a change in appearance (e.g., rhinoplasty, breast augmentation) are more likely to result in a body-image disturbance than restorative procedures designed to restore a body feature to its original state (e.g., rhytidectomy). A recent review of the literature confirmed this finding (Slavin & Beer, 2017). Procedures that result in a change of sensation, such as the feeling of tight skin after a face lift, or the loss of nipple sensation after a breast augmentation, may also influence the client's outcome, with greater degrees of sensory disturbance making it more difficult for the client to view the results positively (Pruzinsky & Edgerton, 1990). In a systematic review of the literature, Herruer, Prins, van Heerbeek, Verhagen-Damen, and Ingels (2015) found there were seven negative predictors for satisfaction in clients undergoing facial cosmetic surgery: 1) male sex, 2) age less than 40 years, 3) unrealistic expectations concerning the surgical result, 4) unrealistic expectations regarding a secondary result (e.g., clients undergoing surgery to improve relationships), 5) minimal deformities, 6) narcissistic personality, and 7) obsessive personality. Notably, clients with psychiatric diseases (e.g., depression, anxiety) and body dysmorphic disorder are more likely to have negative outcomes after plastic or aesthetic procedures (Castle, Honigman, & Phillips, 2002; Slavin & Beer, 2017).

The plastic and aesthetic RN evaluates and applies nursing research findings to promote effective and efficient care and improved client outcomes. The plastic and aesthetic RN works with other members of the healthcare team to identify clinical problems and use existing evidence to improve practice. RNs must demonstrate that nursing interventions make a positive difference in the outcomes and health status of plastic and aesthetic healthcare clients. The plastic and aesthetic RN uses research findings to decrease practice variations, improve outcomes, create standards of excellence for clinical care, and develop practice policies. In addition, the plastic and aesthetic RN assures that practice changes are based on current evidence and, when necessary, seeks out expert resources to assist with implementing the specific steps of EBP. Plastic and aesthetic RNs should seek knowledge and experiences that broaden and maintain current nursing and medical knowledge and evidence relevant to practice.

Increased demand for aesthetic procedures has resulted in a higher number of plastic surgery RNs undertaking the role of aesthetic RN. Many aesthetic treatments and procedures that claim to rejuvenate the skin are not evidence-based; therefore, the plastic and aesthetic RN must review and critically appraise the evidence and utilize only the best evidence and client feedback to guide practice. In this emerging area of practice, the plastic and aesthetic RN generates an ongoing, systematic evaluation of long-term outcomes and implements practice changes as appropriate. There is a need for research in this emerging area of practice, and the plastic and aesthetic RN is positioned to conduct this research. Evidence-based practice undergirds and advances the professional practice of all plastic and aesthetic RNs.

Ethics and Advocacy in Plastic and Aesthetic Nursing

Nursing ethics are based on care and the actions of caring, to enhance and protect the well-being of healthcare clients. Plastic and aesthetic RNs are expected to comply with and promote the ethical ideals, model, code, and principles of the nursing profession. The *Code of Ethics for Nurses with Interpretive Statements* (ANA, 2015b) is the framework on which plastic and aesthetic RNs base ethical analysis and decision-making and on which standards of care are based.

The plastic and aesthetic RN is also an advocate for the healthcare client and provides care in a nondiscriminatory and nonjudgmental manner. Client advocacy mandates preservation of autonomy, execution of clinical judgments, and management of ethical issues. The plastic and aesthetic RN maintains the plastic and aesthetic nursing scope and standards of practice and standards of professional performance in each type of practice environment to help ensure safety, quality of care, and the highest level of health maintenance or health restoration for the client undergoing plastic or aesthetic procedures.

The plastic and aesthetic RN's attitude and performance reflect compassion and respect for the client's cultural beliefs, sovereignty, and right to self-determination and privacy. Plastic and aesthetic RNs implement the principles of autonomy, nonmaleficence, beneficence, and justice when interacting with clients requiring or desiring plastic or aesthetic interventions. The values and obligations in the *Code of Ethics for Nurses* apply to RNs in all roles, in all forms of practice, and in all settings. In fact, it informs every aspect of the RN's life. (ANA, 2015, p. vii)

Plastic and Aesthetic Nursing Explications

The *ANA Code of Ethics for Nurses with Interpretive Statements* (2015) is composed of nine provisions. The ISPAN has provided the Explications for Plastic and Aesthetic Nurses to help plastic and aesthetic RNs incorporate the ANA Code of Ethics into their own practice.

Provision 1.

The nurse practices with compassion and respect for the inherent dignity, worth, and unique attributes of every person.

Explications for Plastic and Aesthetic Nurses

The plastic and aesthetic RN:

- Addresses plastic and aesthetic client concerns compassionately, without bias or judgment.

- Respects the plastic and aesthetic client's autonomy with regard to the provision of informed consent.

- Provides culturally considerate care to the plastic and aesthetic client.

- Respects the plastic or aesthetic client's autonomous decision to undergo plastic or aesthetic procedures.

- Provides nursing care that respects the dignity of the plastic and aesthetic client.

- Applies standards of plastic and aesthetic nursing practice equally to all clients without regard for disability; socioeconomic status; educational level; cultural, religious, or spiritual beliefs; ethnicity; gender identity; sexual orientation; or age.

- Recognizes the value of all members of the plastic and aesthetic healthcare team and treats all members with civility and respect.

Provision 2.

The RN's primary commitment is to the client, whether an individual, family, group, community, or population.

Explications for Plastic and Aesthetic Nurses.

The plastic and aesthetic RN:

- Recognizes the professional nature of the RN-client relationship and adheres to its intrinsic boundaries.

- Promotes treatments that are in the best interest of the plastic and aesthetic client by providing education regarding all available treatment options.

- Collaborates with the plastic and aesthetic healthcare team to plan care specific to the client's needs.

- Acts as an advocate for the plastic and aesthetic client and significant others.

- Campaigns against misleading advertising that sets unrealistic expectations with regard to plastic and aesthetic client outcomes.
- Formulates ethical decisions using available resources (e.g., ethics committee, counselors.)
- Identifies and resolves conflicts of interest.
- Abstains from influencing purchasing decisions that may result in financial gain.
- Does not solicit or accept gifts or gratuities that could be interpreted by others as influencing partiality.

Provision 3.
The nurse promotes, advocates for, and protects the rights, health, and safety of the client.

Explications for Plastic and Aesthetic Nurses.
The plastic and aesthetic RN:

- Restricts access to plastic and aesthetic client care areas to authorized personnel only.
- Avoids needless exposure of the plastic or aesthetic client's body.
- Maintains confidentiality of plastic and aesthetic client information.
- Adheres to federal and state regulations and institutional policies relevant to client rights (e.g., HIPAA, social media, photography consent).
- Refrains from posting images, recordings, or commentary that may breach his or her obligation to maintain and protect the plastic and aesthetic client's privacy.
- Secures the plastic and aesthetic client's records, belongings, and valuables.
- Follows recommended protocols when using investigational devices or participating in new plastic or aesthetic procedures.
- Participates in educational programs that enhance plastic and aesthetic client care.
- Empowers the plastic or aesthetic client with relevant, accurate, and thorough information and education.

- Upholds current standards of evidence-based practice.
- Complies with federal and state regulations related to client safety (e.g., OSHA).
- Follows established protocols for reporting errors.
- Collaborates with facility risk managers and follows organizational policies related to managing errors.
- Questions plastic or aesthetic care that appears inappropriate or substandard.
- Reports incompetent, unethical, or illegal practice accurately and objectively.
- Reports verbal, psychological, and physical harassment or abuse.
- Takes appropriate action to ensure plastic or aesthetic client safety.

Provision 4.

The nurse has authority, accountability, and responsibility for nursing practice; makes decisions; and takes action consistent with the obligation to promote health and to provide optimal care.

Explications for Plastic and Aesthetic Nurses.

The plastic and aesthetic RN:

- Maintains nursing licensure and adheres to state board of nursing regulations.
- Strives to obtain and maintains certification.
- Engages in ongoing continuing education relevant to plastic and aesthetic nursing practice.
- Provides safe and competent plastic and aesthetic client care.
- Questions orders that appear incorrect or inappropriate.
- Accepts responsibility and accountability for his or her plastic or aesthetic nursing practice.
- Consults other healthcare providers for assistance as necessary.
- Protects the scope of RN practice by advocating for and recognizing that only qualified individuals should perform nonsurgical aesthetic procedures.

- Promotes the plastic and aesthetic client's health by providing counseling and recommending specific interventions that promote skin health and can be implemented to impact the client's general overall health.

Provision 5.

The nurse owes the same duties to self as to others, including the responsibility to promote health and safety, preserve wholeness of character and integrity, maintain competence, and continue personal and professional growth.

Explications for Plastic and Aesthetic Nurses.

The plastic and aesthetic RN:

- Practices the same health promotion activities he or she teaches.

- Obtains health care as needed.

- Strives to adhere to healthy life practices including eating a healthy diet, exercising, getting sufficient rest, maintaining healthy relationships, engaging in adequate leisure activities, and attending to spiritual or religious needs.

- Strives to promote and maintain a healthy work life balance

- Implements appropriate safety precautions at all times by utilizing personal protective equipment, laser goggles, smoke evacuation systems, and other safety equipment.

- Attends professional conventions and lectures and reads professional journals pertaining to plastic and aesthetic nursing.

- Maintains accurate records of continuing education and certification activities.

Provision 6.

The nurse, through individual and collective effort, establishes, maintains, and improves the ethical environment of the work setting and conditions of employment that are conducive to safe, quality health care.

Explications for Plastic and Aesthetic Nurses.

The plastic and aesthetic RN:

- Displays empathy, sensitivity, and patience in all aspects of plastic or aesthetic practice, including during stressful or difficult situations.

- Reflects on his or her own virtues, behaviors, and practice to promote personal and professional improvement and growth.

- Participates in developing policies, procedures, and standards of performance for plastic or aesthetic nursing care.

- Assists members of the interprofessional plastic and aesthetic team to practice safely.

- Holds all members of the interprofessional team accountable to high standards of quality in health care.

- Remains alert to changes in the plastic and aesthetic environment that could compromise patient care or safe practice.

Provision 7.

The nurse, in all roles and settings, advances the profession through research and scholarly inquiry, professional standards development, and the generation of both nursing and health policy.

Explications for Plastic and Aesthetic Nurses.

The plastic and aesthetic RN:

- Supports clinical research to examine and develop effective plastic and aesthetic products, procedures, and protocols.

- Uses research findings to support and improve plastic and aesthetic practice.

- Disseminates research findings to colleagues and plastic and aesthetic clients.

- Adheres to plastic and aesthetic investigational device protocols and regulations.

- Advocates for and protects human participants in research occurring in the plastic and aesthetic environment.

- Participates in plastic and aesthetic quality and process improvement initiatives.

- Supports the development of evidence-based position statements, guidelines, and standards for the plastic and aesthetic specialty.

- Supports the generation of advisory statements to clarify the scope of plastic and aesthetic nursing.

Provision 8.

The nurse collaborates with other health professionals and the public to protect human rights, promote health diplomacy, and reduce health disparities.

Explications for Plastic and Aesthetic Nurses.

The plastic and aesthetic RN:

- Collaborates with members of other professional nursing organizations at the state, national, and international levels.
- Collaborates with RNs from other specialties to protect the rights of all clients.
- Communicates knowledge specific to the specialty of plastic and aesthetic nursing to other health professionals.
- Educates members of the community about plastic and aesthetic nursing.
- Advocates for the client's right to plastic and aesthetic care.
- Incorporates the client's cultural differences into the plastic and aesthetic plan of care.
- Incorporates requests for alternative therapies into plastic or aesthetic nursing care and advocates for alternative therapies as appropriate.
- Advocates for human rights in health care.

Provision 9.

The profession of nursing, collectively through its professional organizations, must articulate nursing values, maintain the integrity of the profession, and integrate principles of social justice into nursing and health policy.

Explications for Plastic and Aesthetic Nurses.

The plastic and aesthetic RN:

- Advocates for political representation relevant to plastic and aesthetic nursing at the local, state, and federal level.
- Supports the ISPAN as the specialty's professional organization.
- Recognizes that inequities and personal prejudices adversely affect client outcomes.

- Recognizes the responsibility to intervene with the appropriate persons if it is known that the plastic or aesthetic client is being discharged to an unsafe or unhealthy environment.
- Leads by example to promote equity and social justice.
- Volunteers, as able, to participate in providing community health services.

Insurance Reimbursements

In most cases, insurance plans do not cover the cost of cosmetic procedures and clients undergoing cosmetic procedures must pay out of pocket. Since clients with lower income levels are less able to afford cosmetic procedures, the financial impact is much greater, resulting in socioeconomic disparity.

Insurance coverage for a variety of plastic and aesthetic procedures is highly variable. Although there may be a clear therapeutic benefit and significant improvement in quality of life associated with the procedure, clients may be denied coverage because the insurance company has concluded that the procedure is either cosmetic or not medically necessary (Almazon, Boskey, Labow, & Ganor, 2019; Braun, Braun, Hernandez, & Monson, 2018). Previously, the decision as to whether or not a procedure was medically necessary was made by the surgeon. Currently, there is no clearly established definition of medical necessity; therefore, insurance companies, rather than physicians, are determining eligibility for procedural coverage (Skinner, 2013). Some insurance companies also have additional qualifiers that can negate coverage even when given proof of medical necessity (Rasko et al., 2019).

Almazan et al. (2019), found that insurance coverage for benign breast procedures was highly variable across insurers and procedures. Although reduction mammaplasty, gynecomastia, and gender-affirming mastectomy use similar techniques and share a similar purpose (i.e., to relieve psychological and physical distress caused by excess breast tissue), the variance in coverage suggests that gender may play a role in determining coverage, with men being denied coverage more frequently than women. Men who are candidates for medically necessary surgical correction of gynecomastia are often denied coverage for this procedure (Rasko et al., 2019). Liposuction is an integral part of many gynecomastia procedures; however, some insurance companies may cover the excision portion of the procedure but will not cover the liposuction portion (Rasko et al., 2019). Braun et al. (2018), found that insurance companies consistently denied coverage for reconstructive procedures on pediatric clients with congenital breast anomalies because the surgery was deemed to be cosmetic or not medically necessary.

Post-bariatric body contouring has been shown to improve quality of life and career progression (Al-Hadithy, Hosakere, & Stewart, 2014); yet, there is significant variation in the coverage provided by insurance companies for body contouring surgery for post-bariatric clients. Although cosmetic, these procedures may actually be medically necessary to prevent functional impairment and recurrent skin conditions (Ngaage et al, 2019). Facial feminization surgery is a necessary component of the treatment of gender dysphoria, yet coverage for these procedures is commonly denied by insurers as being cosmetic, or not medically necessary (Dubov & Fraenkel, 2018).

Obtaining reimbursement for plastic and aesthetic procedures is best facilitated by educating insurance providers as to the differences between cosmetic and reconstructive surgery and nonsurgical aesthetic treatments. In the absence of any actual deformity or trauma, cosmetic surgery and aesthetic treatments seek to improve the client's features on a purely aesthetic level. In contrast, the purpose of reconstructive surgery is to correct any physical feature that is grossly deformed or abnormal by accepted standards—either as the result of a birth defect, illness, or trauma. Often, reconstructive surgery not only addresses the deformed appearance, but also seeks to correct or improve some deficiency or abnormality in function as well.

Plastic and aesthetic RNs are in a unique position to act as client advocates or change agents to help secure insurance reimbursements for clients undergoing surgical and nonsurgical procedures. The RN is responsible for providing accurate and thorough documentation. Documenting relevant functional limitations, physical symptoms, and psychological impairments can provide evidence that the procedure is not being performed solely for cosmetic reasons (Braun et al., (2018)

Summary of the Scope of Plastic and Aesthetic Nursing Practice

Plastic and aesthetic nursing specializes in the protection, maintenance, safety, and optimization of health and human bodily restoration and repair before, during, and after cosmetic and reconstructive plastic surgical procedures or nonsurgical aesthetic procedures. The plastic and aesthetic RN collaborates, consults, and serves as a liaison and advocate for individuals, families, groups, communities, and populations. With the dynamic and changing health care practice environment, the plastic and aesthetic RN seeks to utilize the best available evidence and client feedback to guide a holistic practice and promote optimal client outcomes.

Standards of Plastic and Aesthetic Nursing Practice

Standards of Plastic and Aesthetic Nursing Practice

Standard 1. Assessment

The plastic and aesthetic RN collects comprehensive data pertinent to the healthcare client's health and/or situation.

COMPETENCIES

The plastic and aesthetic RN:

▶ Collects data pertinent to the plastic and aesthetic client, including but not limited to demographics, social determinants of health, health disparities, and physical, functional, psychosocial, emotional, cognitive, sexual, cultural, age-related, environmental, spiritual, transpersonal, and economic assessments, in a systematic, ongoing process with compassion and respect for the inherent dignity, worth, and unique attributes of every person.

▶ Recognizes the importance of the assessment parameters identified by Healthy People 2020 (U.S. Department of Health and Human Services, 2018), or other organizations that influence plastic and aesthetic nursing practice.

▶ Integrates knowledge from global and environmental factors into the plastic and aesthetic assessment process.

▶ Elicits the plastic or aesthetic healthcare client's values, preferences, expressed and unexpressed needs, and knowledge of the healthcare situation.

- Recognizes the impact of one's own personal attitudes, values, and beliefs on the plastic and aesthetic assessment process.
- Identifies barriers to effective plastic and aesthetic communication based on psychosocial, literacy, financial, and cultural considerations.
- Assesses the impact of family dynamics on the plastic or aesthetic health care client's health and wellness.
- Engages the plastic or aesthetic health care client and other inter-professional team members in holistic, culturally sensitive data collection.
- Prioritizes data collection based on the plastic or aesthetic healthcare client's immediate condition or the anticipated needs of the healthcare client or situation.
- Uses evidence-based assessment techniques, instruments, tools, available data, information, and knowledge relevant to the plastic or aesthetic situation to identify patterns and variances.
- Applies ethical, legal, and privacy guidelines and policies to the collection, maintenance, use, and dissemination of plastic and aesthetic data and information.
- Recognizes the plastic or aesthetic health care client as the authority on their own health by honoring their healthcare preferences.
- Documents plastic and aesthetic data accurately and in a manner accessible to the interprofessional team.

ADDITIONAL COMPETENCIES FOR THE GRADUATE-LEVEL PREPARED PLASTIC OR AESTHETIC RN

In addition to competencies of the RN, the graduate-level prepared plastic or aesthetic RN:

- Assesses the effect of interactions among plastic and aesthetic individuals, family, community, and social systems on health and illness.
- Synthesizes the plastic and aesthetic results and information leading to clinical understanding.

ADDITIONAL COMPETENCIES FOR THE PLASTIC OR AESTHETIC APRN

In addition to the competencies of the RN and the graduate-level prepared RN, the plastic or aesthetics APRN:

▶ Initiates diagnostic tests and procedures relevant to the plastic or aesthetic healthcare client's current status.

▶ Uses advanced assessment, knowledge, and skills to maintain, enhance, or improve plastic and aesthetic health conditions.

Standard 2. Diagnosis

The plastic and aesthetic RN analyzes assessment data to determine actual or potential diagnoses, problems, and issues.

COMPETENCIES

The plastic and aesthetic RN:

▶ Identifies actual or potential risks to the plastic or aesthetic health-care client's health and safety or barriers to health, which may include but are not limited to interpersonal, systematic, or environmental circumstances.

▶ Uses plastic and aesthetic assessment data, standardized classification systems, technology, and clinical decision support tools to articulate actual or potential diagnoses, problems, and issues.

▶ Verifies the plastic and aesthetic diagnoses, problems, and issues with the individual, family, group, community, population, and interprofessional colleagues.

▶ Prioritizes diagnoses, problems, and issues based on mutually established goals to meet the needs of the plastic or aesthetic health care client across the health-illness continuum.

▶ Documents plastic and aesthetic diagnoses, problems, and issues in a manner that facilitates the determination of the expected outcomes and plan.

ADDITIONAL COMPETENCIES FOR THE GRADUATE-LEVEL PREPARED PLASTIC OR AESTHETIC RN

In addition to the competencies of the RN, the graduate-level prepared plastic or aesthetic RN:

▶ Uses information and communication technologies to analyze plastic and aesthetic diagnostic practice patterns of RNs and other members of the interprofessional health care team.

▶ Employs aggregate-level data to articulate diagnoses, problems, and issues of plastic or aesthetic healthcare clients and organizational systems.

ADDITIONAL COMPETENCIES FOR THE PLASTIC OR AESTHETIC APRN

In addition to the competencies of the RN and the graduate-level prepared RN, the plastic or aesthetic APRN:

▶ Formulates a differential diagnosis based on the plastic or aesthetic assessment, history, physical examination, and diagnostic test results.

Standard 3. Outcomes Identification

The plastic and aesthetic RN identifies expected outcomes for a plan individualized to the healthcare client or the situation.

COMPETENCIES

The plastic and aesthetic RN:

- ▶ Engages the plastic or aesthetic healthcare client, interprofessional team, and others in partnership to identify expected outcomes.
- ▶ Formulates culturally sensitive expected outcomes derived from plastic and aesthetic assessments and diagnoses.
- ▶ Uses clinical expertise and current evidence-based practice to identify plastic and aesthetic health risks, benefits, costs, and/or expected trajectory of the condition.
- ▶ Collaborates with the plastic or aesthetic health care client to define expected outcomes integrating the health care client's culture, values, and ethical considerations.
- ▶ Generates a time frame for the attainment of expected plastic and aesthetic outcomes.
- ▶ Develops expected outcomes that facilitate continuity of plastic and aesthetic care.
- ▶ Modifies expected outcomes based on an evaluation of the status of the plastic or aesthetic health care client and situation.
- ▶ Documents expected outcomes as measurable plastic and aesthetic goals.
- ▶ Evaluates the actual plastic and aesthetic outcomes in relation to expected outcomes, safety, and quality standards.

ADDITIONAL COMPETENCIES FOR THE GRADUATE-LEVEL PREPARED PLASTIC OR AESTHETIC RN, INCLUDING APRN

In addition to the competencies of the RN, the graduate-level prepared plastic or aesthetic RN or APRN:

▶ Defines expected plastic and aesthetic outcomes that incorporate cost and clinical effectiveness and are aligned with the outcomes identified by members of the interprofessional team.

▶ Differentiates plastic and aesthetic outcomes that require care process interventions from those that require system-level actions.

▶ Integrates scientific evidence and best practices to achieve expected plastic and aesthetic outcomes.

▶ Advocates for outcomes that reflect the plastic or aesthetic healthcare client's culture, values, and ethical concerns.

Standard 4. Planning
The plastic and aesthetic RN develops a plan that prescribes strategies to attain expected measurable outcomes.

COMPETENCIES
The plastic and aesthetic RN:

- ▶ Develops an individualized, holistic, evidence-based plan in partnership with the plastic or aesthetic healthcare client and interprofessional team.
- ▶ Establishes the plan priorities with the plastic or aesthetic healthcare client and interprofessional team.
  - ▪ Advocates for responsible and appropriate use of interventions to minimize unwarranted or unwanted treatment and/or plastic or aesthetic healthcare client suffering.
  - ▪ Includes evidence-based strategies in the plan to address each of the identified plastic and aesthetic diagnoses, problems, or issues. These may include but are not limited to
    - ▸ promotion and restoration of health,
    - ▸ prevention of illness, injury, and disease,
    - ▸ facilitation of healing,
    - ▸ alleviation of suffering, and
    - ▸ supportive care.
  - ▪ Incorporates a plastic and aesthetic implementation pathway that describes steps and milestones.
  - ▪ Identifies cost and economic implications of the plastic or aesthetic plan.
  - ▪ Develops a plastic or aesthetic plan that reflects compliance with current statutes, rules and regulations, and standards.
  - ▪ Modifies the plan according to the ongoing assessment of the plastic or aesthetic healthcare client's response and other outcome indicators.
  - ▪ Documents the plastic or aesthetic plan using standardized language or recognized terminology.

ADDITIONAL COMPETENCIES FOR THE GRADUATE-LEVEL PREPARED PLASTIC OR AESTHETIC RN

In addition to the competencies of the RN, the graduate-level prepared plastic or aesthetic RN:

▶ Designs strategies and tactics to meet the multifaceted and complex needs of plastic or aesthetic healthcare clients or others.

▶ Leads the design and development of interprofessional processes to address the identified plastic and aesthetic diagnoses, problems, or issues.

▶ Designs innovative plastic and aesthetic nursing practices.

▶ Actively participates in the development and continuous improvement of plastic and aesthetic systems that support the planning process.

ADDITIONAL COMPETENCIES FOR THE PLASTIC OR AESTHETIC APRN

In addition to the competencies of the RN and the graduate-level prepared RN, the plastic or aesthetic APRN:

▶ Integrates plastic and aesthetic assessment strategies, diagnostic strategies, and therapeutic interventions that reflect current evidence-based knowledge and practice.

▶ Initiates diagnostic tests and procedures relevant to the plastic or aesthetic healthcare client's current status.

▶ Uses advanced assessment, knowledge, and skills to maintain, enhance, or improve plastic and aesthetic health conditions and wellness initiatives.

Standard 5. Implementation
The plastic and aesthetic RN implements the identified plan.

COMPETENCIES
The plastic and aesthetic RN:

▶ Partners with the plastic or aesthetic healthcare client to implement the plan in a safe, efficient, timely, and equitable manner (IOM, 2010).

▶ Integrates interprofessional team partners in implementation of the plastic or aesthetic plan through collaboration and communication across the continuum of care.

▶ Demonstrates caring behaviors to develop therapeutic plastic or aesthetic relationships.

▶ Provides culturally congruent, holistic care that focuses on the plastic or aesthetic healthcare client and addresses and advocates for the needs of diverse populations across the lifespan.

▶ Uses evidence-based interventions and strategies to achieve the mutually identified goals and outcomes specific to the plastic or aesthetic problem or needs.

▶ Integrates critical thinking and technology solutions to implement the nursing process to collect, measure, record, retrieve, trend, and analyze data and information to enhance nursing practice and the plastic or aesthetic healthcare client's outcomes.

▶ Delegates according to the health, safety, and welfare of the plastic or aesthetic healthcare client and considering the circumstance, person, task, direction or communication, supervision, evaluation, as well as the state RN practice act regulations, institution, and regulatory entities while maintaining accountability for the care.

▶ Documents implementation and any modifications, including changes or omissions, of the identified plastic or aesthetic plan.

ADDITIONAL COMPETENCIES FOR THE GRADUATE-LEVEL PREPARED PLASTIC OR AESTHETIC RN

In addition to the competencies of the RN, the graduate-level prepared plastic or aesthetic RN:

► Uses systems, organizations, and community resources to lead effective change and implement the plastic or aesthetic plan.

► Applies quality principles while articulating methods, tools, performance measures, and standards as they relate to implementation of the plastic and aesthetic plan.

► Translates plastic and aesthetic evidence into practice.

► Leads plastic and aesthetic interprofessional teams to communicate, collaborate, and consult effectively.

► Demonstrates plastic and aesthetic leadership skills that emphasize ethical and critical decision-making, effective working relationships, and a systems perspective.

► Serves as a plastic and aesthetic consultant to provide additional insight and potential solutions.

► Uses theory-driven plastic and aesthetic approaches to effect organizational or system change.

ADDITIONAL COMPETENCIES FOR THE PLASTIC OR AESTHETIC APRN

In addition to the competencies of the RN and the graduate-level prepared RN, the plastic or aesthetic APRN:

► Uses plastic and aesthetic prescriptive authority, procedures, referrals, treatments, and therapies in accordance with state and federal laws and regulations.

► Prescribes traditional and integrative evidence-based treatments, therapies, and procedures that are compatible with the plastic or aesthetic healthcare client's cultural preferences and norms.

► Prescribes evidence-based pharmacological agents and treatments according to plastic and aesthetic clinical indicators and results of diagnostic and laboratory tests.

► Provides clinical consultation for plastic or aesthetic healthcare clients and professionals related to complex clinical cases to improve care and client outcomes.

Standard 5A. Coordination of Care

The plastic and aesthetic RN coordinates care delivery.

COMPETENCIES

The plastic and aesthetic RN:

- ▶ Organizes the components of the plan.
- ▶ Collaborates with the plastic or aesthetic client to help manage health care based on mutually agreed upon outcomes.
- ▶ Manages a plastic or aesthetic healthcare client's care in order to reach mutually agreed upon outcomes.
- ▶ Engages plastic or aesthetic healthcare clients in self-care to achieve preferred goals for quality of life.
- ▶ Assists the plastic or aesthetic healthcare client to identify options for care.
- ▶ Advocates for the delivery of dignified and holistic care by the inter-professional team.
- ▶ Documents the coordination of the plastic or aesthetic care.
- ▶ Provides leadership in the coordination of interprofessional heath care for integrated delivery of plastic or aesthetic healthcare client care services to achieve safe, effective, efficient, timely, client-centered, and equitable plastic or aesthetic care (IOM, 2010).

ADDITIONAL COMPETENCIES FOR THE PLASTIC OR AESTHETIC APRN

In addition to the competencies of the RN, the plastic or aesthetic APRN:

- ▶ Manages identified plastic or aesthetic client panels or populations.
- ▶ Serves as the plastic or aesthetic healthcare client's primary care provider and coordinator of health care services in accordance with state and federal laws and regulations.
- ▶ Synthesizes plastic or aesthetic data and information to prescribe and provide necessary system and community support measures, including modifications of environment.

Standard 5B. Health Teaching and Health Promotion

The plastic and aesthetic RN employs strategies to promote health and a safe environment.

COMPETENCIES

The plastic and aesthetic RN:

▶ Provides opportunities for the plastic or aesthetic healthcare client to identify needed health care promotion, disease prevention, and self-management topics.

▶ Uses health promotion and health teaching methods in collaboration with the plastic or aesthetic healthcare client's values, beliefs, health practices, developmental level, learning needs, readiness and ability to learn, language preference, spirituality, culture, and socioeconomic status.

▶ Uses feedback and evaluations from the plastic or aesthetic healthcare client to determine the effectiveness of the employed strategies.

▶ Uses technologies to communicate health promotion and disease prevention information to the plastic or aesthetic healthcare client.

▶ Provides plastic or aesthetic healthcare clients with information about intended effects and potential adverse effects of the plan of care.

▶ Engages client alliance and advocacy groups in health teaching and health promotion activities for plastic or aesthetic healthcare clients.

▶ Provides anticipatory guidance to plastic or aesthetic healthcare clients to promote health and prevent or reduce the risk of negative health outcomes.

ADDITIONAL COMPETENCIES FOR THE GRADUATE-LEVEL PREPARED AND PLASTIC OR AESTHETIC APRN

In addition to the competencies of the RN, the graduate-level prepared or plastic or aesthetic APRN:

▶ Synthesizes empirical evidence on risk behaviors, gender roles, learning theories, behavioral change theories, motivational theories, translational theories for evidence-based practice, epidemiology, and other related theories and frameworks when designing plastic or aesthetic health education information and programs.

▶ Evaluates health information resources for applicability, accuracy, readability, and comprehensibility to help plastic or aesthetic healthcare clients access quality health information.

▶ Evaluates health information resources, such as the Internet, within the area of plastic and aesthetic nursing practice for accuracy, readability, and comprehensibility, to help healthcare clients access quality health information.

▶ Engages client alliances and advocacy groups, as appropriate, in plastic or aesthetic health teaching and health promotion activities.

▶ Provides anticipatory guidance to individuals, families, groups, and communities to promote health and prevent or reduce the risk of plastic or aesthetic health problems.

Standard 6. Evaluation

The plastic or aesthetic RN evaluates progress toward attainment of goals and outcomes.

COMPETENCIES

The plastic or aesthetic RN:

▶ Conducts a holistic, systematic, ongoing, and criterion-based evaluation of the outcomes in relation to the structure, processes, and timeline prescribed in the plan.

▶ Collaborates with the plastic or aesthetic healthcare client and others involved in the care or situation in the evaluation process..

▶ Determines, in partnership with the plastic or aesthetic healthcare client and other stakeholders, the client-centeredness, effectiveness, efficiency, safety, timeliness, and equitability (IOM, 2001) of the strategies in relation to the responses to the plan and attainment of outcomes. Other defined criteria (e.g., Quality and Safety Education for Nurses) may be used as well.

▶ Uses ongoing assessment data to revise the diagnoses, outcomes, plan, and implementation strategies

▶ Documents the results of the evaluation.

ADDITIONAL COMPETENCIES FOR THE GRADUATE-LEVEL PREPARED AND PLASTIC OR AESTHETIC APRN

In addition to the competencies of the RN, the graduate-level prepared plastic or aesthetic APRN:

▶ Evaluates the accuracy of the diagnosis and effectiveness of the interventions and other variables in relation to the plastic or aesthetic healthcare client's attainment of expected outcomes.

▶ Adapts the plan of care for the trajectory of treatment according to the evaluation of response.

▶ Synthesizes evaluation data from the plastic or aesthetic healthcare client, community, population and/or institution to determine the effectiveness of the plan.

▶ Engages in a systematic evaluation process to revise the plan to enhance its effectiveness.

▶ Uses results of the evaluation to make or recommend process, policy, procedure, or protocol revisions when warranted.

Standards of Professional Performance for Plastic and Aesthetic Nursing

Standard 7. Ethics

The plastic or aesthetic RN practices ethically.

COMPETENCIES

The plastic or aesthetic RN:

▶ Integrates the *Code of Ethics for Nurses with Interpretive Statements* (ANA, 2015b) to guide nursing practice and articulate the moral foundation of nursing.

▶ Practices with compassion and respect for the inherent dignity, worth, and unique attributes of all people.

▶ Advocates for plastic or aesthetic healthcare clients' rights to informed decision-making and self-determination.

▶ Seeks guidance in situations where the rights of the individual conflict with public health guidelines.

▶ Endorses the understanding that the primary commitment is to the plastic or aesthetic healthcare client regardless of setting or situation.

▶ Maintains therapeutic and professional boundaries.

▶ Advocates for the rights, health, and safety of the plastic or aesthetic healthcare client and others.

▶ Safeguards the privacy and confidentiality of plastic or aesthetic healthcare clients, others, and their data and information within ethical, legal, and regulatory parameters.

▶ Demonstrates professional accountability and responsibility for nursing practice.

▶ Maintains competence through continued personal and professional development.

▶ Demonstrates commitment to self-reflection and self-care.

▶ Contributes to the establishment and maintenance of an ethical environment that is conducive to safe, quality health care.

► Advances the profession through scholarly inquiry, professional standards development, and the generation of policy.

► Collaborates with other health professionals and the public to protect human rights, promote health diplomacy, enhance cultural sensitivity and congruence, and reduce health disparities.

► Articulates nursing values to maintain personal integrity and the integrity of the profession.

► Integrates principles of social justice into nursing and policy.

Standard 8. Culturally Congruent Practice

The plastic or aesthetic RN practices in a manner that is congruent with cultural diversity and inclusion principles.

COMPETENCIES

The plastic or aesthetic RN:

▶ Demonstrates respect, equity, and empathy in actions and interactions with all healthcare clients.

▶ Participates in life-long learning to understand cultural preferences, worldview, choices, and decision-making processes of diverse clients.

▶ Creates an inventory of one's own values, beliefs, and cultural heritage.

▶ Applies knowledge of variations in health beliefs, practices, and communication patterns in all nursing practice activities.

▶ Identifies the stage of the plastic and aesthetic client's acculturation and accompanying patterns of needs and engagement.

▶ Considers the effects and impact of discrimination and oppression on practice within and among vulnerable cultural groups.

▶ Uses skills and tools that are appropriately vetted for the culture, literacy, and language of the population served.

▶ Communicates with appropriate language and behaviors, including the use of medical interpreters and translators in accordance with client preferences.

▶ Identifies the cultural-specific meaning of the interactions, terms, and content.

▶ Respects client decisions based on age, tradition, belief and family influence, and stage of acculturation.

▶ Advocates for policies that promote health and prevent harm among culturally diverse, under-served, or under-represented clients.

▶ Promotes equal access to services, tests, interventions, health promotion programs, enrollment in research, education, and other opportunities.

▶ Educates RN colleagues and other professionals about cultural similarities and differences of healthcare clients, families, groups, communities, and populations.

ADDITIONAL COMPETENCIES FOR THE GRADUATE-LEVEL PREPARED PLASTIC OR AESTHETIC RN

In addition to the competencies of the RN, the graduate-level prepared plastic or aesthetic RN:

► Evaluates tools, instruments, and services provided to culturally diverse populations.

► Advances organizational policies, programs, services, and practice that reflect respect, equity, and values for diversity and inclusion.

► Engages plastic or aesthetic clients, key stakeholders, and others in designing and establishing internal and external cross-cultural partnerships.

► Conducts research to improve plastic or aesthetic health care and health care outcomes for culturally diverse clients.

► Develops recruitment and retention strategies to achieve a multicultural workforce.

ADDITIONAL COMPETENCIES FOR THE PLASTIC OR AESTHETIC APRN

In addition to the competencies of the RN and the graduate-level prepared RN, the plastic or aesthetic APRN:

► Promotes shared decision-making solutions in planning, prescribing, and evaluating processes when the plastic or aesthetic healthcare client's cultural preferences and norms may create incompatibility with evidence-based practice.

► Leads interprofessional teams to identify the cultural and language needs of the plastic or aesthetic client.

Standard 9. Communication

The plastic or aesthetic RN communicates effectively in all areas of practice.

COMPETENCIES

The plastic or aesthetic RN:

▶ Assesses one's own communication skills and effectiveness.

▶ Demonstrates cultural empathy when communicating.

▶ Assesses communication ability, health literacy, and resources of plastic or aesthetic healthcare clients to inform the interprofessional team and others.

▶ Uses language translation resources to ensure effective communication.

▶ Incorporates appropriate alternative strategies to communicate effectively with plastic or aesthetic healthcare clients who have visual, speech, language, or communication difficulties.

▶ Uses communication styles and methods that demonstrate caring, respect, deep listening, authenticity, and trust.

▶ Conveys accurate information.

▶ Maintains communication with interprofessional team and others to facilitate safe transitions and continuity in care delivery.

▶ Contributes the plastic or aesthetic nursing perspective in interactions with others and discussions with the interprofessional team.

▶ Exposes care processes and decisions when they do not appear to be in the best interest of the plastic or aesthetic healthcare client.

▶ Discloses concerns related to potential or actual hazards and errors in care or the practice environment to the appropriate level.

▶ Demonstrates continuous improvement of communication skills.

ADDITIONAL COMPETENCIES FOR THE GRADUATE-LEVEL PREPARED AND PLASTIC OR AESTHETIC APRN

In addition to the competencies of the RN, the graduate-level prepared plastic or aesthetic RN or plastic or aesthetic APRN:

▶ Assumes a leadership role in shaping or fashioning environments that promote healthy communication.

Standard 10. Collaboration

The plastic or aesthetic RN collaborates with the healthcare client, family, and others in the conduct of plastic and aesthetic nursing practice.

COMPETENCIES

The plastic or aesthetic RN:

- ▶ Identifies the areas of expertise and contribution of other professionals and key stakeholders.
- ▶ Clearly articulates the RN's role and responsibilities within the team.
- ▶ Partners with the plastic or aesthetic healthcare client and key stakeholders to advocate for and effect change, leading to positive outcomes and quality care.
- ▶ Uses appropriate tools and techniques, including information systems and technologies, to facilitate discussion and team functions, in a manner that protects dignity, respect, privacy, and confidentiality.
- ▶ Promotes engagement through consensus building and conflict management.
- ▶ Uses effective group dynamics and strategies to enhance team performance.
- ▶ Exhibits dignity and respect with interacting with others and giving and receiving feedback.
- ▶ Partners with all stakeholders to create, implement, and evaluate a comprehensive plan.

ADDITIONAL COMPETENCIES FOR THE GRADUATE-LEVEL PREPARED AND PLASTIC OR AESTHETIC APRN

In addition to the competencies of the RN, the graduate-level prepared plastic or aesthetic APRN:

- ▶ Participates in interprofessional activities, including, but not limited to education, consultation, management, technological development, or research to enhance outcomes.

- ▶ Provides leadership for establishing, improving, and sustaining collaborative relationships to achieve safe, quality care for plastic or aesthetic healthcare clients.

- ▶ Advances interprofessional plan-of-care documentation and communications, rationales for plan-of-care changes, and collaborative discussions to improve plastic or aesthetic healthcare client outcomes.

Standard 11. Leadership

The plastic and aesthetic RN leads within the professional practice setting and in the profession.

COMPETENCIES

The plastic and aesthetic RN:

► Contributes to the establishment of an environment that supports and maintains respect, trust, and integrity.

► Encourages innovation in practice and role performance to attain personal and professional plans, goals, and vision.

► Communicates to manage change and address conflict.

► Mentors colleagues for the advancement of plastic and aesthetic nursing practice and the profession to enhance safe, quality health care.

► Retains accountability for delegated nursing care.

► Contributes to the evolution of the plastic and aesthetic nursing profession through participation in professional organizations.

► Influences policy to promote health.

► Advocates for the healthcare client's right to pursue elective plastic and aesthetic procedures and treatments.

ADDITIONAL COMPETENCIES FOR THE GRADUATE-LEVEL PREPARED AND PLASTIC OR AESTHETIC APRN

In addition to the competencies of the RN, the graduate-level prepared or plastic or aesthetic APRN:

► Influences decision-making bodies to improve the professional practice environment and plastic and aesthetic healthcare client outcomes.

► Enhances the effectiveness of the interprofessional team.

► Promotes advanced practice nursing and role development by interpreting its role for plastic and aesthetic healthcare clients and policy makers.

▶ Models expert practice for interprofessional team members and health care clients.

▶ Mentors colleagues in the acquisition of clinical knowledge, skills, abilities, and judgment related to plastic and aesthetic nursing.

Standard 12. Education

The plastic and aesthetic RN attains knowledge and competence that reflect current plastic and aesthetic nursing practice and promote futuristic thinking.

COMPETENCIES

The plastic and aesthetic RN:

▶ Identifies learning needs based on nursing knowledge and the various roles the plastic and aesthetic RN may assume.

▶ Participates in ongoing educational activities related to nursing and interprofessional knowledge bases and professional topics.

▶ Mentors RNs new to their roles for the purpose of ensuring successful enculturation, orientation, and emotional support.

▶ Demonstrates a commitment to lifelong learning through self-reflection and inquiry for learning and personal growth.

▶ Seeks experiences that reflect current plastic and aesthetic nursing practice, to maintain and advance knowledge, skills, abilities, and judgment in clinical practice or role performance.

▶ Pursues training and apprenticeship opportunities to expand knowledge and skills related to plastic and aesthetic nursing practice.

▶ Acquires knowledge and skills relative to the role, population, specialty, setting, and global or local health situation.

▶ Identifies modifications or accommodations needed in the delivery of education based on plastic and aesthetic healthcare client and family members' needs.

▶ Participates in formal or informal consultations to address issues in plastic and aesthetic nursing practice as an application of education and knowledge.

▶ Shares educational findings, experiences, and ideas with peers.

▶ Supports acculturation of plastic and aesthetic RNs new to their roles by role modeling, encouraging, and sharing pertinent information relative to optimal care delivery.

▶ Facilitates a work environment supportive of ongoing education of plastic and aesthetic health care professionals.

▶ Maintains a professional portfolio that provides evidence of individual competence and lifelong learning.

Standard 13. Evidence-Based Practice and Research

The plastic and aesthetic RN integrates evidence and research findings into practice.

COMPETENCIES

The plastic and aesthetic RN:

- ▶ Articulates the values of research and its application relative to the health care setting and practice.
- ▶ Identifies questions in the plastic and aesthetic health care setting and practice that can be answered by nursing research.
- ▶ Uses current evidence-based nursing knowledge, including research findings, to guide practice.
- ▶ Incorporates evidence when initiating changes in plastic and aesthetic nursing practice.
- ▶ Participates in the formulation of evidence-based practice through research.
- ▶ Promotes ethical principles of research in plastic and aesthetic nursing practice and the health care setting.
- ▶ Appraises nursing research for optimal application in plastic and aesthetic nursing practice and the health care setting.
- ▶ Shares peer reviewed research findings with colleagues to integrate knowledge into plastic and aesthetic nursing practice.
- ▶ Supports the publication of a professional nursing journal specific to plastic and aesthetic nursing practice.

ADDITIONAL COMPETENCIES FOR THE GRADUATE-LEVEL PREPARED AND PLASTIC OR AESTHETIC APRN

In addition to the competencies of the RN, the graduate-level prepared or plastic or aesthetic APRN:

- ▶ Integrates research-based practice in all plastic and aesthetic settings.
- ▶ Uses current health care research findings and other evidence to expand knowledge, skills, abilities, and judgment; to enhance role performance; and to increase knowledge of professional plastic and aesthetic issues.

- ▶ Uses critical thinking skills to connect theory and research to plastic and aesthetic practice.
- ▶ Integrates nursing research to improve quality in plastic and aesthetic nursing practice.
- ▶ Contributes to plastic and aesthetic nursing knowledge by conducting or synthesizing research and other evidence that discovers, examines, and evaluates current practice, knowledge, theories, criteria, and creative approaches to improve health care outcomes.
- ▶ Encourages other plastic and aesthetic RNs to develop research skills.
- ▶ Performs rigorous critique of evidence derived from databases to generate meaningful evidence for plastic and aesthetic nursing practice.
- ▶ Advocates for the ethical conduct of research and translational scholarship with particular attention to the protection of the plastic and aesthetic health care client as a research participant.
- ▶ Promotes a climate of collaborative research and clinical inquiry.
- ▶ Disseminates research findings through activities such as presentations, publications, consultation, and journal clubs.

Standard 14. Quality of Practice

The plastic and aesthetic RN contributes to quality nursing practice.

COMPETENCIES

The plastic and aesthetic RN:

▶ Ensures that plastic and aesthetic nursing practice is safe, effective, efficient, equitable, timely, and client-centered (IOM, 1999; IOM, 2001).

▶ Identifies barriers and opportunities to improve health care safety, effectiveness, efficiency, equitability, timeliness, and client-centeredness.

▶ Recommends strategies to improve plastic and aesthetic nursing quality.

▶ Uses creativity and innovation to enhance plastic and aesthetic nursing care.

▶ Participates in quality improvement activities

▶ Collects data to monitor the quality of plastic and aesthetic nursing practice.

▶ Provides critical review and/or evaluation of policies, procedures, and guidelines to improve the quality of health care.

▶ Engages in formal and informal peer review processes.

▶ Collaborates with the interprofessional team to implement quality improvement plans and interventions.

▶ Documents plastic and aesthetic nursing practice in a manner that supports quality and performance improvement initiatives.

▶ Achieves professional certification in plastic and/or aesthetic nursing.

ADDITIONAL COMPETENCIES FOR THE GRADUATE-LEVEL PREPARED PLASTIC OR AESTHETIC RN

In addition to the competencies of the RN, the graduate-level prepared plastic or aesthetic RN:

► Analyzes trends in plastic and aesthetic health care quality data, including examination of cultural influences and factors.

► Conducts regular reviews of client outcomes to identify potential areas of opportunity for quality improvement initiatives.

► Incorporates evidence into nursing practice to improve outcomes.

► Designs innovations to improve client outcomes.

► Provides leadership in the design and implementation of quality improvement initiatives.

► Promotes a practice environment that supports evidence-based health care.

► Contributes to nursing and interprofessional knowledge through scientific inquiry.

► Encourages professional or specialty certification.

► Engages in development, implementation, evaluation, and/or revision of policies, procedures, and guidelines to improve health care quality.

► Uses data and information in system-level decision-making.

► Influences the organizational system to improve client outcomes.

ADDITIONAL COMPETENCIES FOR THE PLASTIC OR AESTHETIC APRN

In addition to the competencies of the RN and the graduate-level prepared RN, the plastic or aesthetic APRN:

► Engages in comparison evaluations of the efficacy and effectiveness of diagnostic tests, clinical procedures, products and therapies, and treatment plans, in partnership with healthcare clients, to optimize health and healthcare quality.

► Designs quality improvement studies, research initiatives, and programs to improve health outcomes in diverse settings where plastic and aesthetic nursing care is provided.

▶ Applies knowledge obtained from advanced preparation, as well as current research and evidence-based information, to clinical decision-making at the point of care to achieve optimal health outcomes.

▶ Uses available benchmarks as a means to evaluate practice at the individual, departmental, or organizational level.

Standard 15. Professional Practice Evaluation

The plastic and aesthetic RN evaluates one's own and others' nursing practice.

COMPETENCIES

The plastic and aesthetic RN:

▶ Engages in self-reflection and self-evaluation of plastic and aesthetic nursing practice on a regular basis, identifying areas of strength as well as areas in which professional growth would be beneficial.

▶ Adheres to the guidance about professional practice as specified in the *Nursing: Scope and Standards of Practice* and the *Code of Ethics for Nurses with Interpretive Statements*.

▶ Ensures that nursing practice is consistent with regulatory requirements pertaining to licensure, relevant statutes, rules, and regulations.

▶ Uses organizational policies and procedures to guide professional practice.

▶ Incorporates recommendations from the professional plastic and aesthetic nursing organizational body into professional practice.

▶ Influences organizational policies and procedures to promote inter-professional evidence-based practice.

▶ Provides the evidence for practice decisions and actions as part of the informal and formal evaluation processes.

▶ Seeks formal and informal feedback regarding one's own plastic and aesthetic nursing practice from healthcare clients, peers, colleagues, supervisors, and others.

▶ Provides peers and others with formal or informal constructive feedback regarding their practice and role performance.

▶ Takes action to achieve goals identified during the evaluation process.

Standard 16. Resource Utilization

The plastic and aesthetic RN utilizes appropriate resources to plan, provide, and sustain evidence-based nursing services that are safe, effective, and fiscally responsible.

COMPETENCIES

The plastic and aesthetic RN:

- ▶ Assesses plastic and aesthetic healthcare client care needs and resources available to achieve desired outcomes.

- ▶ Assists the plastic and aesthetic healthcare client in factoring costs, risks, and benefits in decisions about care.

- ▶ Assists the plastic and aesthetic healthcare client in identifying and securing appropriate services to address needs across the health care continuum.

- ▶ Delegates in accordance with applicable legal and policy parameters.

- ▶ Identifies impact of resource allocation on the potential for harm, complexity of the task, and desired outcomes.

- ▶ Advocates for resources that support and enhance plastic and aesthetic nursing practice.

- ▶ Integrates telehealth and mobile health technologies into practice to promote positive interactions between plastic and aesthetic health care clients and care providers.

- ▶ Uses organizational and community resources to implement interprofessional plans for the plastic and aesthetic client.

- ▶ Addresses discriminatory health care practices and the impact on resource allocation.

- ▶ Examines protocols and procedures for potential misuse of resources and/or unnecessary waste generation.

ADDITIONAL COMPETENCIES FOR THE GRADUATE-LEVEL PREPARED PLASTIC OR AESTHETIC RN

In addition to the competencies of the RN, the graduate-level prepared plastic or aesthetic RN:

▶ Designs innovative solutions to use resources effectively and maintain quality.

▶ Creates evaluation strategies that address cost effectiveness, cost benefit, and efficiency factors associated with nursing practice.

▶ Assumes complex and advanced leadership roles to initiate and guide change.

▶ Encourages members of the interprofessional team to utilize resources thoughtfully and effectively.

ADDITIONAL COMPETENCIES FOR THE PLASTIC OR AESTHETIC APRN

In addition to the competencies of the RN and the graduate-level prepared RN, the plastic or aesthetic APRN:

▶ Engages organizational and community resources to formulate and implement interprofessional plans.

Standard 17. Environmental Health

The plastic and aesthetic RN practices in an environmentally safe and healthy manner.

COMPETENCIES

The plastic and aesthetic RN:

▶ Promotes a safe and healthy workplace and professional practice environment.

▶ Uses environmental health concepts in practice.

▶ Assesses the environment to identify risk factors.

▶ Reduces environmental health risks to self, colleagues, and health-care clients.

▶ Communicates information about environmental health risks and exposure reduction strategies.

▶ Encourages members of the interprofessional team to take owner-ship of the health of the practice environment.

▶ Advocates for the safe, judicious, and appropriate use and disposal of products in health care.

▶ Incorporates technologies to promote safe practice environments.

▶ Uses products or treatments consistent with evidence-based practice to reduce environmental threats.

▶ Participates in developing strategies to promote health communities and practice environments.

ADDITIONAL COMPETENCIES FOR THE GRADUATE-LEVEL PREPARED AND PLASTIC OR AESTHETIC APRN

In addition to the competencies of the RN, the graduate-level prepared or plastic or aesthetic APRN:

▶ Analyzes the impact of social, political, and economic influences on the global environment and human health experience.

▶ Creates partnerships that promote sustainable global environmental health policies and conditions that focus on prevention of hazards to people and the natural environment (ANA, 2007).

Glossary

Advanced Practice Registered Nurse (APRN). Advanced Practice RNs include nurse practitioners, clinical nurse specialists, nurse anesthetists, and nurse midwives. These nurses are often primary care providers. Advanced Practice RNs treat and diagnose illnesses, advise the public on health issues, manage chronic disease, and engage in ongoing education to stay current with technological, methodological, or other developments in the field. In addition to the initial nursing education and licensing required for all RNs, APRNs hold at least a master's degree.

Aesthetic. A specialty encompassing procedures aimed at improving or restoring the physical appearance and satisfaction of the client, utilizing surgical or nonsurgical modalities.

Body dysmorphic disorder. A disorder characterized by intense preoccupation with an imagined defect in appearance. This disorder is observed in approximately 7% to 15% of cosmetic surgery clients (Higgins & Wysong, 2018). The illness begins in adolescence and affects men and women equally.

Body image. A personal perception of one's physical appearance based on self-observation, emotions, physical sensations, and the reactions of others.

Clinical Nurse Specialist. An APRN trained to provide expert advice related to specific conditions or treatment pathways.

Dermatology. A branch of medicine dealing with the function and diseases of the skin, nails, and hair.

Ear gauging. A piercing of the earlobe that is gradually expanded over a period of years by inserting piercings of incrementally larger sizes to increase the diameter of the dilated ear holes. Also known as ear stretching or ear plugging.

Holism (holistic). A view of everything in terms of patterns and processes that combine to form a whole, instead of seeing things as fragments, pieces, or parts. Holistic nursing embraces nursing practice where healing the whole person is the goal. Holism involves understanding the individual as an integrated whole interacting with and being acted upon by both internal and external environments.

Interdisciplinary. Relating to, or using a combination of, several disciplines for a common purpose. An interdisciplinary team is a unit composed of individuals with varied and specialized expertise who coordinate their activities to provide services to patients with an actual or potential diagnosis. The team engages in collaborative endeavors using the combined skills and expertise of team members. The patient is a member of the team whenever possible and appropriate.

Intraoperative phase. Begins when the client enters the operating or procedure room and ends when the client enters the post anesthesia care unit.

Multimodal analgesia. The use of two or more pharmacologic or nonpharmacologic interventions to reduce pain.

Nurse Practitioner. An APRN trained to assess client needs, order and interpret diagnostic and laboratory tests, diagnose illness and disease, prescribe medication, and formulate treatment plans.

Oculoplastics. A branch of medicine and surgery that includes a wide variety of surgical procedures dealing with the eye socket, eyelids, tear ducts, and the face. It also deals with the reconstruction of the eye and associated structures.

Ophthalmology. A branch of medicine and surgery that deals with the diagnosis and treatment of eye disorders.

Otorhinolaryngology. A branch of medicine and surgery that deals with the head and neck, ear, nose, and throat.

Perioperative. A term used to describe the three phases of any surgical procedure: preoperative, intraoperative, and postoperative.

Plastic. A specialty encompassing surgical techniques and treatment strategies for human body and facial repair, reconstruction, and replacement in cases of congenital deformities or diseases, traumatic injuries, and removal of tissue due to cancer or disease.

Preoperative phase. Begins with the decision to have surgery and ends when the client enters the operating or procedure room.

Postoperative phase. The period immediately following surgery. This phase can be brief, lasting one to a few hours, or require months of rehabilitation and recuperation.

Standard. An authoritative statement enunciated and promulgated by the profession, by which the quality of practice, service, or education can be judged.

Tattoo. A type of body art that marks human skin with indelible designs by introducing exogenous pigment into the dermis using a needle or other sharp object laden with pigment until the image is created. Tattoos can also occur accidentally (e.g., shotgun blast, road surface trauma).

References

Al-Hadithy, N., Hosakere, A., & Stewart, K. (2014). Does the degree of ptosis predict the degree of psychological morbidity in bariatric patients undergoing reconstruction? *Plastic and Reconstructive Surgery, 134*(5), 942–950.

Almazon, A. N., Boskey, E. R., Labow, B., & Ganor, O. (2019). Insurance policy trends for breast surgery in cisgender women, cisgender men, and transgender men. Plastic and Reconstructive Surgery, Advance online publication. http://doi.org/10.1097/PRS.0000000000005852

American Association of Colleges of Nursing. (2011). The essentials of master's education in nursing. Available at https://www.aacnnursing.org/Portals/42/Publications/Masters Essentials11.pdf

American Board of Medical Specialties (ABMS). (2000). *Member boards and associate members.* Available at https://www.abms.org/member-boards/

American Nurses Association (ANA). (2007). *ANA principles of environmental health for nursing practice with implementation strategies.* Silver Spring, MD: Nursesbooks.org.

American Nurses Association (ANA). (2010). *Nursing's social policy statement: The essence of the profession.* Silver Spring, MD: Nursesbooks.org.

American Nurses Association (ANA). (2015a). *Nursing: Scope and standards of practice* (3rd ed.). Silver Spring, MD: ANA.

American Nurses Association (ANA). (2015b). *Code of ethics for nurses with interpretive statements* (2nd ed.). Silver Spring, MD: ANA.

American Society of periAnesthesia Nurses (ASPAN). (2018). *Perianesthesia nursing standards, practice recommendations, and interpretive statements, 2019-2020.* Cherry Hill, NJ: ASPAN.

Association of periOperative Registered Nurses (AORN). (2019). *Guidelines for perioperative practice.* Denver, CO: AORN, Inc.

Association of periOperative Registered Nurses (AORN). (2015). *Standards of perioperative nursing.* Available at https://www.aorn.org/guidelines/clinical-resources/aorn-standards

American Society for Aesthetic Plastic Surgery. (2019). *Guidelines for patients seeking cosmetic procedures.* Available at https://www.surgery.org/consumers/consumer-resources/consumer-tips/guidelines-for-patients-seeking-cosmetic-procedures-abroad

American Society of Plastic Surgeons. (2012). *ASPS cautions plastic surgery patients to approach holiday medical tourism with vigilance.* Available at https://www.plasticsurgery.org/news/press-releases/asps-cautions-plastic-surgery-patients-to-approach-holiday-medical-tourism-with-vigilance

American Society of Plastic Surgeons. (2018). *New trends survey shows plastic surgeons eager for future advances to meet growing consumer demands.* Available at https://www.plasticsurgery.org/news/press-releases/new-trends-survey-shows-plastic-surgeons-eager-for-future-advances-to-meet-growing-consumer-demands

American Society of Plastic Surgeons. (2019). *Plastic surgery statistics.* Available at https://www.plasticsurgery.org/news/plastic-surgery-statistics

Berli, J.U., Knudson, G., Fraser, L., Tangpricha, V., Etner, R., Ettner, F.M., . . . Schechter, Ll. (2017). What surgeons need to know about gender confirmation surgery when providing care for transgender individuals: A review. *JAMA Surgery, 152*(4), 394–400.

Braun, T. L., Braun, J. L., Hernandez, C., & Monson, L. A. (2018). Insurance appeals for pediatric reconstructive surgery. *Annals of Plastic Surgery, 80*(3), 198-204.

Brennan, C. (2018). The art of the consultation experience. *Plastic Surgical Nursing, 38*(1), 35–40.

Castle, D. J., Honigman, R. J., & Phillips, K. A. (2002). Does cosmetic surgery improve psychosocial wellbeing? *Medical Journal of Australia, 176*(12), 601–604.

Dubov, A., & Fraenkel, L. (2018). Facial feminization surgery: The ethics of gatekeeping in transgender health. *American Journal of Bioethics, 18*(12), 3–9.

Edgerton, M. T., Jacobsen, W. E., & Meyer, E. (1960). Surgical-psychiatric study of patients seeking plastic (cosmetic) surgery: Ninety-eight consecutive patients with minimal deformity. *British Journal of Plastic Surgery, 13*, 136–145.

Farley, C. L., Van Hoover, C., & Rademeyer, C. A. (2019). Women and tattoos: Fashion, meaning, and implications for health. *Journal of Midwifery & Women's Health, 64*(2), 154–169.

Garcia-Vilarino, E., Salmeron-Gonzalez, E., Perez-Garcia, A., Ruiz-Cases, A., Condino-Brito, E., & Sanchez-Garcia, A. (2018). Forequarter amputation, thoracic resection, and reconstruction on giant ulcer due to locally advanced oncological disease. *Plastic Surgical Nursing, 38*(3), 128–132.

Gart, M. S. (2014). Pediatric plastic surgery: Four-dimensional medicine. *Plastic Surgical Nursing, 34*(1), 23–24.

Glass, J. S., Hardy, C. L., Meeks, N. M., & Carroll, B. T. (2015). Acute pain management in dermatology: Risk assessment and treatment. *Journal of the American Academy of Dermatology, 73*(4), 543–560.

Glatt, B. S., Sarwer, D. B., O'Hara, D. E., Hamori, C., Bucky, L. P., & LaRossa, D. (1999). A retrospective study of changes in physical symptoms and body image after reduction mammaplasty. *Plastic and Reconstructive Surgery, 103*(1), 76–85.

Hass, C. F., Champion, A., & Secor, D. (2008). Motivating factors for seeking cosmetic surgery. *Plastic Surgical Nursing, 28*(4), 177–182.

Heike, C.L., Leavitt, D., Aspinall, C., Andrews, M., Carey, H., & Ose, M. (2010). Craniofacial summer camp: An educational experience for campers, camp staff, and the craniofacial team. *Plastic Surgical Nursing, 30*(1), 6–11.

Henderson, J., & Malata, C. M. (2010). Surgical correction of the expanded earlobe after ear gauging. *Aesthetic Plastic Surgery, 34*(5), 632–633.

Herruer, J. M., Prins, J. B., van Heerbeek, N., Verhage-Damen, G. W. J. A., & Ingels, K. J. A. O. (2015). Negative predictors for satisfaction in patients seeking facial cosmetic surgery: A systematic review. *Plastic and Reconstructive Surgery, 135*(6), 1596–1605.

Higgins, S., & Wysong, A. (2018). Cosmetic surgery and body dysmorphic disorder—An update. *International Journal of Women's Dermatology, 4*(1), 43–48.

Ho, S. G., & Goh, C. L. (2015). Laser tattoo removal: A clinical update. *Journal of Cutaneous Aesthetic Surgery, 8*(1), 9–15.

Institute of Medicine (IOM). (2001). *Crossing the quality chasm.* Washington, DC: National Academies Press.

Institute of Medicine (IOM). (2010). *The future of nursing: Leading change, advancing health.* Washington, DC: National Academies Press.

International Society of Plastic and Aesthetic Nursing (ISPAN). (2018). *Position statement on laser, light, and energy therapy.* Retrieved from http://ispan.org/multimedia/files/position-statements/Laser-Light-Therapy.pdf

International Society of Plastic and Aesthetic Nursing (ISPAN). (2019). *PSN: Language and editing services.* Retrieved from https://journals.lww.com/psnjournalonline/_layouts/15/1033/oaks.journals/editservices.aspx

Islam, P. S., Chang, C., Selmi, C., Generali, E., Huntley, A., Teuber, S. S., & Gershwin, M. E. (2016). Medical complications of tattoos: A comprehensive review. *Clinical Reviews in Allergy & Immunology, 50*(2), 273–286.

LoGiudice, J., & Gosain, A. K. (2004). Pediatric tissue expansion: Indications and complications. *Plastic Surgical Nursing, 24*(1), 20–26.

Ngaage, L. M., Rose, J., Pace, L., Kambouris, A. R., Rada, E. M., Kligman, M. D., & Rasko, Y. M. (2019). A review of national insurance coverage of post-bariatric upper body lift. *Aesthetic Plastic Surgery.* Advance online publication. http://doi.org/10.1007/s00266-019-01420-7

Pek, W. S., Goh, L. H. T., & Pek, C. H. (2017). The rolling earlobe flap for dilated ear holes following ear gauging: A novel approach to aesthetically preserving earlobe soft tissue volume. *Archives of Plastic Surgery, 44*(5), 453–456.

Pruzinsky, T., Edgerton, M. T. (1990). Body-image change in cosmetic plastic surgery. In T. F. Cash, & T. Pruzinsky (Eds.), *Body images: Development, deviance, and change* (pp. 217–236). New York, NY: Guildford Press.

Rankin, M., & Mayers, P.M. (2008). Core curriculum for plastic surgical nursing: Psychosocial care of the plastic surgical patient. *Plastic Surgical Nursing, 28*(1), 12–24.

Rasko, Y. M., Rosen, C., Ngaage, L. M., Cantab, M. B., AlFadil, S., Elegbede, Al, . . . Slezak, S. (2019). Surgical management of gynecomastia: A review of the current insurance coverage criteria. *Plastic and Reconstructive Surgery, 143*(5), 1361–1368.

Ross, K. M., Moscoso, A. V., Bayer, L. R., Rosselli-Risal, L., & Orgill, D. P. (2018). Plastic surgery complications from medical tourism treated in a U.S. academic medical center. *Plastic and Reconstructive Surgery, 141*(4), 517e–523e.

Rudolph, R., & Miller, S. (2000). Reconstruction after Mohs' cancer excision. *Plastic Surgical Nursing, 20*(3), 186.

Sarwer, D. B., Wadden, T. A., Pertschuk, M. J., & Whitaker, L. A. (1998). Body image dissatisfaction and body dysmorphic disorder in 100 cosmetic surgery patients. *Plastic and Reconstructive Surgery, 101*(6), 1644–1649.

Shannon-Missal, L. (2018). Tattoo takeover: Three in ten Americans have tattoos, and most don't stop at just one. *The Harris Poll* website. Available at https://theharrispoll.com/tattoos-can-take-any-number-of-forms-from-animals-to-quotes-to-cryptic-symbols-and-appear-in-all-sorts-of-spots-on-our-bodies-some-visible-in-everyday-life-others-not-so-much-but-one-thi/

Sidner, S. (2017). Old mark of slavery is being used on sex trafficking victims. *CNN News* website. Available at https://www.cnn.com/2015/08/31/us/sex-trafficking-branding/index.html

Skinner, D. (2013). Defining medical necessity under the patient protection and affordable care act. *Public Administration Review, 73*(s1), S49–S59.

Slavin, B., & Beer, J. (2017). Facial identity and self-perception: An examination of psychosocial outcomes in cosmetic surgery patients. *Journal of Drugs in Dermatology, 16*(6), JO0617.

Snell, B. J., & Caplash, Y. (2013). A novel way to repair the earlobe after ear gauging. *Journal of Plastic & Aesthetic Surgery, 66*(1), 140–148.

Steffen, L.E., Johnson, A. Levine, B.J., Mayer, D.K., & Avis, N.E. (2017). Met and unmet expectations for breast reconstruction in early posttreatment breast cancer survivors. *Plastic Surgical Nursing, 37*(4), 146–153.

Sullivan, M. A., & Adkinson, J.M. (2016). Congenital hand differences. *Plastic Surgical Nursing, 36*(2), 84–89.

Survivor's Ink. (2017). From victim to survivor. *CNN Freedom Project* website. Available at https://www.cnn.com/2015/08/31/us/sex-trafficking-branding/index.html

Svientek, S., & Levine, J. (2015). Pediatric burns of the hand. *Plastic Surgical Nursing, 35*(2), 81–82.

U.S. Department of Health and Human Services. (2018). *Healthy people 2020.* Available at https://www.healthypeople.go

Wakefield, W., Rubin, J. P., & Gusenoff, J. A. (2014). The life after weight loss program: A paradigm for plastic surgery care after massive weight loss. *Plastic Surgical Nursing, 34*(1), 4–9.

Wang, Q., Cao, C., Guo, R., Xiaoge, L., Lu, L., Wang, W., & Li, S. (2016). Avoiding psychological pitfalls in aesthetic medical procedures. *Aesthetic Plastic Surgery, 40*(6), 954–961.

Appendix A
Plastic Surgery Nursing: Scope and Standards of Practice (2013)

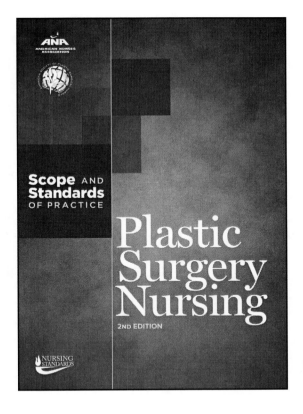

Scope AND
Standards
OF PRACTICE

Plastic Surgery Nursing

2ND EDITION

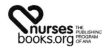

American Nurses Association
Silver Spring, Maryland
2013

Contents

iii

Contributors

Scope and Standards Task Force

Sharon Fritzsche, RN, MSN, APRN-BC

Judy Akin, MSN, RN, PHN

Marcia Spear, DNP, ACNP-BC, CWS, CPSN

Patricia M. Terrell, MSN, CPNP, CNOR, CPSN

Jacqueline Frazee, BSN, CNOR, RNFA, CPSN

Claudette J. Heddens, MA, BSN, ARNP, CPSN

Stephanie Dinman, MSN, CRNP, FNP

Christine Brajkovich, BSN, CNOR, RNFA, CPSN

Michelle Rooks, RN

Special thanks to the Clinical Practice Committee Chairman Sharon D. Fritzsche, MSN, RN, APRN-BC, and committee member Judy Akin, MSN, RN, PHN, of the ASPSN for initiating and completing the process of having the ASPSN recognized as a specialty organization by the ANA. Also, a special thanks to the Scope and Standards Task Force members for their work on updating and presenting the new edition of the Scope and Standards of Practice for Plastic Surgery Nursing. The ASPSN would also like to give thanks to Carol J. Bickford, PhD, RN-BC, CPHIMS Senior Policy Fellow, Department of Nursing Practice and Policy, for her guidance and reference in the updates and revisions of the Scope of Practice Statement and revision of the Standards of Practice and Professional Performance for the ASPSN.

v

The content in this appendix is not current and is of historical significance only.

CONTRIBUTORS

American Nurses Association (ANA) Staff

Carol Bickford, PhD, RN-BC, CPHIMS—Content editor

Maureen E. Cones, Esq.—Legal counsel

Yvonne Daley Humes, MSA—Project coordinator

Eric Wurzbacher, BA—Project editor

About the American Nurses Association

The American Nurses Association (ANA) is the only full-service professional organization representing the interests of the nation's 3.1 million registered nurses through its constituent/state nurses associations and its organizational affiliates. The ANA advances the nursing profession by fostering high standards of nursing practice, promoting the rights of nurses in the workplace, projecting a positive and realistic view of nursing, and by lobbying the Congress and regulatory agencies on health care issues affecting nurses and the public.

About the American Society of Plastic Surgical Nurses

The American Society of Plastic Surgical Nurses (ASPSN) is committed to the enhancement of quality nursing care delivered to the patient undergoing plastic and reconstructive surgery and nonsurgical aesthetic procedures. ASPSN promotes high standards of plastic and reconstructive surgical and aesthetic nursing practice and patient care through education, analysis and dissemination of information, and scientific inquiry.

About Nursesbooks.org, The Publishing Program of ANA

Nursesbooks.org publishes books on ANA core issues and programs, including ethics, leadership, quality, specialty practice, advanced practice, and the profession's enduring legacy. Best known for the foundational documents of the profession on nursing ethics, scope and standards of practice, and social policy, Nursesbooks.org is the publisher for the professional, career-oriented nurse, reaching and serving nurse educators, administrators, managers, and researchers as well as staff nurses in the course of their professional development.

Scope of Plastic Surgery Nursing Practice

Definition of Plastic Surgery Nursing

Plastic surgery nursing specializes in the protection, maintenance, safety, and optimization of health and human bodily restoration and repair before, during, and after plastic surgery cosmetic, reconstructive, and nonsurgical aesthetic procedures. This is accomplished through the nursing process, and includes diagnosis and treatment of human response. The plastic surgery nurse collaborates, consults, and serves as a liaison and advocate for individuals, families, communities, and populations, bridging the role of the plastic surgery nurse with that of other professionals to promote optimal patient outcomes for the whole person.

Foundation of Plastic Surgery Nursing Practice

The specialty of plastic surgery has long pioneered surgical techniques and treatment strategies for human body and facial repair, reconstruction, and replacement in cases of congenital diseases, traumatic injuries, and cancer reconstruction. Plastic surgery sites include the skin, breast, trunk, craniomaxillofacial structures, musculoskeletal system, extremities, and external genitalia. Plastic surgery focuses on the care of complex wounds, replants, grafts, flaps, free tissue transfer, use of implantable materials, and the healing process and response. In addition, cosmetic or aesthetic surgery is an essential component of plastic surgery and is used both to improve overall appearance and to optimize the outcome of reconstructive procedures. (American Board of Plastic Surgery [ABPS], 2011). Plastic surgery interventions encompass all ages, from the neonate to the advanced geriatric healthcare consumer. This requires specialized knowledge and treatment to ensure optimal outcomes.

1

Plastic surgery is the only specialty recognized and supported by the American Board of Medical Specialties (ABMS, 2000) that provides plastic, reconstructive, and aesthetic surgical procedures through board certification for plastic surgery (www.abms.org).

Media coverage to the general public has deluged our society with information about plastic surgery that is often questionable and confusing. Unfortunately, because of extensive media coverage of plastic surgery and increasing demands for aesthetic plastic surgery, procedures are being performed by other medical specialties without proper preparation, recognition, regulation, board certification, or surgical residency experience. This lack of regulation, specialized knowledge, and skill exposes individuals, families, communities, and populations to unnecessary health and safety risks. Both the increasing awareness in our society (accurate and otherwise) of plastic surgery and the ambiguities of cosmetic surgery call for more nursing, consumer, and provider educational interventions by plastic surgery nurses to help clarify misconceptions. Plastic surgery nurses are aware of the health risks associated with plastic surgery procedures and, as members of the interprofessional healthcare team, complement the plastic surgery specialty by a mutual focus on healthcare consumer safety, health maintenance, and ultimate satisfaction and outcomes.

Plastic surgery nursing practice and standards reflect the nursing process, the nursing standards of both the American Nurses Association (ANA, 2010a) and the Association of periOperative Registered Nurses (AORN) standards of perioperative practice, and AORN standards of nursing practice (AORN, 2011). Plastic surgery nursing requires specialized knowledge and skill levels for both the reconstructive and aesthetic aspects of surgical interventions during the consultation, preoperative, operative, and postoperative stages of the plastic surgery procedure process. Through the implementation and maintenance of specialized plastic surgery nursing standards of practice, individuals seeking or requiring plastic surgery intervention will be provided with education, knowledge, and care to ensure optimal surgical safety, protection, and outcomes.

Development of Plastic Surgery Nursing Practice

Plastic surgery nursing opportunities continue to expand as the demand for plastic surgery procedures and treatments grows, primarily in the United States. According to the American Society of Plastic Surgeons (www.asps .org), more than 17 million plastic surgery procedures and treatments were

Appendix A. Plastic Surgery Nursing: Scope and Standards of Practice (2013)

The content in this appendix is not current and is of historical significance only.

performed in 2009, compared to approximately 1.5 million in 1992. The need for knowledge regarding safety, quality, ethical, and procedural issues will increase as plastic surgery becomes more common in a wide range of surgical environments.

Plastic surgery is an interprofessional specialty. The plastic surgeon's expertise can be utilized by any modality, including but not limited to pediatrics, general surgery, neurosurgery, urology, dermatology, and trauma. Because of the physical and psychological complexities involved in caring for those undergoing plastic surgery, plastic surgery nurses integrate a holistic approach into the plan of care for the plastic surgery healthcare consumer. Plastic surgery nursing skills and knowledge require a strong foundation in the knowledge of pre-, intra-,and postoperative standards and practices; wound healing and wound care; safety and quality; bioethics; psychology; and the application of critical thinking.

In response to the specialized needs of plastic surgery healthcare consumers and the required nursing interventions, 100 surgical nurses convened in 1975 to establish the nonprofit organization called the American Society of Plastic and Reconstructive Surgical Nurses (ASPRSN). In 2001 ASPRSN simplified its name to American Society of Plastic Surgical Nurses (ASPSN). The 100 charter members sought to establish a specialized identity and share the knowledge needed to practice successfully. The mission and philosophy of the ASPSN were founded on principles aimed at improving the quality of nursing care for the healthcare consumer undergoing plastic or reconstructive surgery. The organization is committed to promoting high standards of nursing care and practice through shared knowledge, scientific inquiry, and continuing education, while supporting and encouraging collaborative interaction with clinical practice, administration, research, and academics (www.aspsn.org). The chronology of the development of plastic surgery nursing is summarized below.

Plastic Surgery Nursing: A Chronology

1975   The American Society of Plastic and Reconstructive Surgical Nurses (ASPRSN) held its first national meeting in Toronto, Canada. Sherill Lee Schultz is the first president and founder.

1976   Thirteen local chapters of ASPRSN are established in the United States and Canada.

1980   ASPRSN creates *Plastic Surgical Nursing Journal.*

1980	ASPRSN becomes the 22nd member of the National Federation for Specialty Nursing Organizations.
1984	The plastic surgical nursing bibliography is completed.
1989	The first edition of *Core Curriculum for Plastic and Reconstructive Surgical Nursing* is published. The Plastic Surgical Nursing Certification Board (PSNCB) is established.
1991	The first plastic surgical nursing certification examination (CPSN) is given.
1995	ASPRSN establishes a Research Committee to assist ASPRSN nurses with research funds and priorities unique to plastic surgical nursing practice.
1996	The second edition of *Core Curriculum for Plastic and Reconstructive Surgical Nursing* is published.
1998	ASPRSN creates a website: www.aspsn.org.
2001	ASPRSN simplifies its name to the American Society of Plastic Surgical Nurses (ASPSN).
2004	The specialty is recognized and the ASPSN–ANA specialty standards document, *Plastic Surgery Nursing: Scope and Standards of Practice*, is drafted.
2005	*Plastic Surgery Nursing: Scope and Standards of Practice* is published by ANA.
2007	Third edition of *Core Curriculum for Plastic Surgical Nursing* is published.
2010	Task force is initiated to develop an aesthetic nursing certification.
2010	Workgroup is convened to review and revise *Plastic Surgery Nursing: Scope and Standards of Practice*.

Today the ASPSN has more than 1,000 active members working in various nursing environments: surgical facilities, home care, nursing research, outpatient care, hospitals, universities, private practice, medical or medi-spas, and others. Members cover a wide range of educational levels, including associate, bachelor's, master's, and/or doctorate degrees, and have numerous roles, including advanced practice nurses, nurse first-assistant, and nurse educators. ASPSN serves its members through a national structure of local chapters in the United States and Canada (ASPSN, 2010). Through the development of unique plastic surgery knowledge, the plastic surgery nurse can properly respond to and communicate with a multidisciplinary team assigned to any plastic surgery healthcare consumer.

As the field of plastic surgery evolves and incorporates other medical specialties, the climate for plastic surgery nursing requires continual review of related trends, products, and procedures. Current statistical data found on the American Society of Plastic Surgeon's web site (www.asps.org) for 2009, include a 10% increase in breast reconstruction from 2000 to 2009, with tissue expander reconstruction seeing a 12% increase from 2008 to 2009. Breast reduction surgery has increased by 7% from 2000. Tumor removal, including skin cancers, has decreased from 578,161 procedures in 2000 to 487,146 in 2009. Cosmetic surgical procedures have experienced an overall decline since 2000, with a 20% total decrease. Breast augmentation remains the number-one cosmetic procedure, followed by rhinoplasty. With more and more healthcare consumers undergoing bariatric or weight-loss surgical procedures, the number of body contouring procedures (such as buttock lifts, lower body lifts, and thigh and arm lifts) is increasing significantly, and has experienced more than a 50% increase since 2000 (www.asps.org). Minimally invasive procedures have increased 99% since 2000, with Botox showing a 509% increase from 2000; in addition, there has been a significant rise in procedures for dermal fillers and laser resurfacing (www.asps.org). Due to this extraordinary growth, there has been an influx of nurses into this highly challenging arena of plastic surgery practice.

One goal of plastic surgery nursing is to secure the foundation for safety. This is accomplished through stronger regulations, increased education, and awareness among healthcare consumers, families, communities, and populations seeking or requiring plastic surgery-related interventions.

Plastic surgery nurses promote and improve quality of care before, during, and after plastic surgical procedures and treatments to ensure proper health maintenance, safety, and restoration. Plastic surgery nurses determine the specific nursing intervention needed for each individual undergoing a plastic surgical procedure or treatment, in accordance with the nursing process (assessment, diagnosis, outcomes identification, planning, implementation, and evaluation). This nursing specialty continues to develop the knowledge base for evidence-based practice through research into plastic surgery procedures, treatments, and issues.

Healthcare Consumer Population

The plastic surgery nurse interacts with and cares for healthcare consumers who require or desire plastic or reconstructive surgery for enhancement or restoration purposes. The plastic surgery nurse also interacts with wand educates families of plastic surgery healthcare consumers, as well as communities, regarding plastic surgery procedures and issues. The plastic surgery nurse has the special knowledge and skills needed to meet the needs of the healthcare consumer population. The plastic surgery nurse provides care in a variety of settings, age groups, and populations, including neonatal, pediatric, adult, geriatric, general surgery, neurosurgery, advanced wound management, dermatology, burns, cancer, and trauma healthcare consumers.

Healthcare consumers receiving care and education from a plastic surgery nurse need a thorough understanding of procedures, personal expectations, and mutual goal setting in order to achieve maximum satisfaction and health maintenance. Plastic surgery nurses help healthcare consumers to deal with perceived or altered body image, perceived surgical outcomes, fears, and learning needs associated with a surgical intervention. Healthcare consumers undergoing plastic surgery may encounter psychological, emotional, and physical imbalances during the recovery phase. Managing the psychological discord associated with physical alterations requires specialized knowledge and education.

Reconstructive Plastic Surgery Population

Reconstructive plastic surgery procedures are performed on skin, breast, trunk, craniomaxillofacial structures, musculoskeletal system, extremities, and external genitalia. Nurses in reconstructive plastic surgery require specialized knowledge related to complex wounds, replants, grafts, flaps, free tissue transfer, and use of implantable materials for reconstruction or repair due to cancer, trauma, burns, superficial injury, congenital defects, or disease. Plastic surgery nurses help the patient to express psychological, physical, and psychosocial needs in order to regain or rediscover coping strategies and successful interactions with society. Thorough assessment and documentation before, during, and after surgery is essential for proper evaluation of healthcare consumer outcomes.

Aesthetic Plastic Surgery Population

The plastic surgery nurse must possess a thorough knowledge of anatomy, body systems, operative standards, and the psychological aspects of body image and perception. An understanding of the needs and assessment of expectations places the plastic surgery nurse in the forefront as an advocate for the aesthetic healthcare consumer's safety. Aesthetic plastic surgery procedures may be applied to skin, breast, trunk, craniomaxillofacial structures, musculoskeletal system, extremities, and external genitalia. Aesthetic plastic surgery may be performed after reconstructive surgery to improve overall results. Aesthetic surgery includes adjustment, enhancement, and alteration according to each individual healthcare consumer's request and need for plastic surgery intervention. Thorough assessment and documentation before, during, and after surgery is essential for proper evaluation of patient outcomes.

With the development and introduction of new products and technologies, the quest to defy the aging process and enhance beauty continues. According to the 2008 *Plastic Surgery Procedural Statistics* (American Society of Plastic Surgeons, 2009), there has been a steady increase in the number of consumers who have undergone nonsurgical aesthetic procedures, notably injections of botulinum toxin Type A and dermal fillers. This phenomenon has required that healthcare providers adapt to these technical developments to meet the needs of the population, and has led to increased specialization in the area of plastic surgery nursing. In short, plastic surgery nurses require specialized knowledge associated with reconstructive surgical principles to assist in the successful recovery and outcomes of the aesthetic surgery healthcare consumer.

Roles of Plastic Surgery Nurses

Nursing: Scope and Standards of Practice, Second Edition (ANA, 2010a), *Nursing's Social Policy Statement: The Essence of the Profession* (ANA, 2010b), and *Code of Ethics for Nurses with Interpretive Statements* (ANA, 2001) provide the foundation for all registered nurses and their professional practice. The roles of the plastic surgery nurse further derive from the specialty's scope-of-practice statement and specific standards of care, required educational guidelines, and practice environments and settings serving the plastic surgery healthcare consumer. One of the goals of plastic surgery nursing is to reach and educate other nurses and nursing students about plastic surgery issues, procedures, and current trends. Communication and interaction with other nursing specialties about the role of plastic surgery nurses will provide a broader understanding and knowledge base for nursing collaboration. Plastic surgery nurses help build the foundations of knowledge and education for improved outcomes, safety, health maintenance, and health awareness.

General Nursing Role

Registered nurses beginning clinical practice in their first year of licensure are encouraged to gain knowledge and develop skill levels associated with basic medical and surgical principles in preparation for later specialization in plastic surgery nursing. Registered nurses who enter the field of plastic surgery must have a well-rounded knowledge base about a wide variety of healthcare consumer

Plastic Surgery Nursing: Scope and Standards of Practice 2nd Edition   7

populations. The scope of knowledge required for the plastic surgery nurse varies with the area of practice interest, previous nursing experience, and level of educational preparation. The general-level plastic surgery nurse will progress into a more expert role with experience, training, mentoring, and additional education.

Advanced Practice Role

Advanced practice plastic surgery nursing roles are increasing in response to personal, professional, and societal needs. Nurse practitioner (NP) and clinical nurse specialist (CNS) are two of the roles included in the term *advanced practice*.

Advanced practice registered nurses (APRNs) play a significant role in meeting the needs of the plastic surgery healthcare consumer. APRNs in plastic surgery are valuable in practice because of their ability to use independent judgment in clinical decision-making and to provide skilled, quality, and detailed advanced nursing care across the continuum. An APRN in plastic surgery has the knowledge and training to provide comprehensive health assessments, differential diagnoses, and treatments for plastic surgery healthcare consumers. The APRN in plastic surgery is an advocate for health maintenance, health promotion, and wellness.

Advanced practice registered nurses in plastic surgery serve as resources and consultants to other healthcare disciplines. Legislation has now made prescriptive authority and third-party reimbursement possible for the APRN in the plastic surgery arena. The APRN is instrumental in facilitating and conducting research in plastic surgery and plays a key role in providing continuity of care for the plastic surgery healthcare consumer based on the best evidence. The roles of the APRN in plastic surgery are developing and expanding.

Educator Role

Plastic surgery nurse educators promote educational clarity, standards, knowledge, and safety related to plastic surgery procedures, issues, and outcomes with other nurses, students, healthcare consumers, other providers, and the community. In this document, the plastic surgery registered nurse (RN) in an educator role is referred to as the *plastic surgery nurse educator*.

Even though all nurses are educators in their role of caring for healthcare consumers, a plastic surgery nurse educator is educated at the master's-degree level or higher with a focus on plastic surgery education. A plastic surgery nurse educator requires a strong knowledge base regarding teaching and learning theories, curriculum development, research, test and measurement evaluation methods, critical thinking skills, and quality improvement techniques. Plastic surgery nurse educators also comply with and support state educational requirements to teach at community or university institutions. At the graduate or doctoral level, the plastic surgery nurse educator has the opportunity to facilitate and develop focused education, curriculums, and research in plastic surgery nursing.

A plastic surgery nurse educator conducts a needs assessment to help establish educational requirements in various practice environments and settings. A plastic surgery nurse educator functions as an educator and a liaison between the plastic surgeon or advanced practice registered nurse and the healthcare consumer to help ensure continuity of care, health promotion, and health maintenance. A plastic surgery nurse educator provides an appropriate climate for learning, and ensures that the learners are actively involved in the learning process. The plastic surgery nurse educator collects and analyzes data to evaluate the effectiveness and outcomes of various educational strategies, and, if necessary, provides a revised plan to address shortcomings and problems.

A plastic surgery nurse educator is a member of an interprofessional team, and functions as a consultant, change agent, leader, and resource to other nursing and healthcare disciplines. Plastic surgery nurse educators help to generate research and disseminate findings into education and practice.

A plastic surgery nurse educator, in collaboration with plastic surgery nurses, develops instructions, guidelines, materials, and programs for nurses during nursing school rotations, distance learning experiences, and in various practices, environments, and settings related to plastic surgery. A plastic surgery nurse educator also provides education for local and national communities on plastic surgery and relevant resources.

Specialized Nursing Role

Because the demand for procedures to maintain a youthful appearance and beauty has exploded, the development of new and improved aesthetic nonsurgical technologies, products, and procedures has also grown. This has facilitated the development of the aesthetic nurse role within plastic surgical nursing. With the increasing demand for these procedures, the role of the aesthetic nurse becomes more important in plastic surgery as well as other specialties. The aesthetic nurse has a scope of knowledge more specialized to nonsurgical aesthetic procedures and this population of healthcare consumers than the general plastic surgery nurse, and has undergone additional education and training in anatomy, procedural techniques, products, technologies, assessment, and education specific to the aesthetic nonsurgical healthcare consumer.

The aesthetic nurse must be focused on maintaining the highest standards within the specialty by undergoing continuing education, providing excellent outcomes, and maintaining an unrivaled ethical environment. The aesthetic nurse must always consider the healthcare consumer's specific requests, budget, lifestyle, and expectations. The aesthetic nonsurgical healthcare consumer often hears about new products or procedures via the popular media, so the aesthetic nurse, as a professional, must guide and educate the patient to select an appropriate product, procedure, or technology and make necessary referrals to the physician. As these procedures are out-of-pocket expenses to the individual, the aesthetic nurse has an obligation to recommend and provide only those procedures that are appropriate and to avoid any financial conflict of interest.

Educational Preparation for Plastic Surgery Nursing

Broad experience in surgical duties, sterile technique, and postanesthesia care enhances the ability to build on the skill sets needed for specialty practice. As there are no formal academic educational programs for plastic surgery nursing, plastic surgical nurses must build on the general knowledge and education of their respective nursing programs. The plastic surgery nurse learns plastic surgery fundamentals from professional courses offered by ASPSN, core curriculum materials, mentoring, and seminars and workshops pertaining to plastic surgery education, procedures, and issues. Education, experience, and increased familiarity with plastic surgery procedures and outcomes will increase knowledge and help attain the skill levels needed to care for the plastic surgery healthcare consumer. Due to the complexities of plastic surgery, including psychological and psychosocial factors, plastic surgery nurses require a minimum of two years of experience before seeking certification in plastic surgery nursing.

Minimum Requirements for Plastic Surgery Nursing

- Licensure as a registered nurse within the designated state of practice
- Education:
  - Minimum requirement: Associate's degree from an accredited college of nursing
  - Preferred: Bachelor of science degree in nursing from an accredited college of nursing

- Advanced knowledge in surgical principles, anatomy, and physiology for specified age groups from neonates to older adults
- Advanced knowledge in one or more of the following:
  - Wound care, burns, trauma, cancer-related disfigurements
  - Scar management, body image, health assessment, nutrition
- Continuing education and knowledge of current plastic surgery trends, issues, and procedures
- Certification:
  Plastic surgery nursing certification is available (http://psncb.org/)
- Advanced knowledge and training in anatomy, including muscles and blood vessels, aging, assessment, and technologies (aesthetic role).

Plastic Surgery Nursing Research and Evidence-Based Practice

Evidence-based practice (EBP) is a scholarly and systematic problem-solving paradigm that results in the delivery of high-quality health care. To make the best clinical decisions using EBP, research findings are blended with internal evidence—including practice-generated data, clinical expertise, and healthcare consumer values and preferences—to achieve the best outcomes for individuals, groups, populations, and healthcare systems.

Nursing research and EBP contribute to the body of knowledge and enhance healthcare consumer outcomes. The plastic surgery nurse continually evaluates and applies nursing research findings to promote effective and efficient care and improved outcomes. The plastic surgery nurse works with other members of the healthcare team to identify clinical problems and uses existing evidence to improve practice. Nurses must demonstrate that nursing interventions make a positive difference in the outcomes and health status of plastic surgery healthcare consumers. The plastic surgery nurse uses research findings to decrease practice variations, improve outcomes, and create standards of excellence for care and policies. In addition, the plastic surgery nurse assures that changes made in practice are based on the current evidence and seeks out expert resources to assist with specific steps in EBP. Plastic surgery nurses utilize evidence-based practice to keep abreast of medical knowledge relevant to practice and ensure that they are current and up-to-date on the latest evidence.

Plastic Surgery Nursing: Scope and Standards of Practice 2nd Edition   11

Increased demand for aesthetic procedures has resulted in a higher number of plastic surgery nurses undertaking the role of aesthetic nurse. Many aesthetic treatments and procedures that claim to rejuvenate the skin are not supported by good scientific evidence; therefore, the plastic surgery nurse must critically appraise the evidence and utilize only the best evidence to guide practice. In this emerging area of practice, the plastic surgery nurse generates an ongoing, systematic evaluation of long-term outcomes and implements practice changes as appropriate. There is a need for unbiased funding of research in this emerging area of practice, and the plastic surgery nurse is positioned to seek this funding.

EBP undergirds and advances the professional practice of all plastic surgery nurses. Plastic surgery nurses must be able to gain, assess, apply, and integrate new knowledge, as well as the ability to adapt to changing circumstances and environments.

Practice Environments and Settings for the Plastic Surgery Nurse

The plastic surgery nurse provides care for healthcare consumers and their families or caretakers in a variety of settings and locations that include hospitals, outpatient ambulatory surgery centers, office-based surgery centers, private practice, and newly evolving medical spas. The plastic surgery nurse is prepared to educate and provide comprehensive care to healthcare consumers in a safe and regulated environment. The plastic surgery nurse provides competent, ethical, and appropriate nursing care to help improve surgical experiences and outcomes. To determine and implement the plan of care, and to ensure optimal outcomes for the plastic surgery healthcare consumer, the plastic surgery nurse encourages and facilitates consultations, communication, and collaboration with other healthcare team members. As a healthcare provider, the value and benefit of the APRN in plastic surgery practices are widely recognized, and the APRN is being utilized in many or most of the previously mentioned practice settings and locations.

Plastic surgery nurses are also knowledgeable about proper policies, procedures, contracts, and regulations, including those for compliance with the Health Insurance Portability and Accountability Act (HIPAA), in appropriate and designated plastic surgery settings. Plastic surgery nurses know and comply with the requirements for federal, state, local, insurance, and accreditation agency standards, regardless of the area of practice. Plastic surgery nurses help promote safer surgical services for the plastic surgery healthcare consumer. Regulatory factors pertinent to plastic surgery nurses working in any environment may include The Joint Commission (TJC); the Centers for Medicare and Medicaid Services (CMS); Occupational Safety and Health Administration (OSHA) standards for bloodborne pathogens and hazardous waste; the Americans with Disabilities Act; specific hospital rules and regulations; and rules, regulations, and guidelines established by each state board of nursing. All of these ensure public safety. The plastic surgery nurse should also know and address, as appropriate, compliance with the guidelines of the Accreditation Association for Ambulatory Health Care (AAAHC), the AAAHC Institute for Quality Improvement (IQI), the American Association for Accreditation of Ambulatory Surgery Facilities, Inc. (AAAASF), and the U.S. Food and Drug Administration regarding tissue tracking and drug and/or implant recalls.

Hospitals

The plastic surgery nurse working in the hospital environment may care for plastic surgery healthcare consumers in a variety of specialty departments or units. These include, among others, emergency departments; operating rooms; surgical, burn, critical care, and neonatal units; pediatrics; and oncology. Plastic surgery nursing within the hospital environment is multidimensional and includes skills, functions, roles, and responsibilities that evolve from the body of knowledge specific to plastic surgery nursing. The plastic surgery nurse practicing in the hospital environment may provide assessment, analysis, diagnosis, planning, implementation, interventions, outcome identification, and evaluation of healthcare consumers in all age groups whose care requires plastic surgery interventions, procedures, wound care, and other treatments.

Outpatient/Ambulatory Surgery Centers

The plastic surgery nurse working in the outpatient/ambulatory surgery center demonstrates the appropriate skills, knowledge, competencies, and abilities to provide proper and safe nursing care for the plastic surgery healthcare consumer in the preoperative, operative, and postoperative stages of the plastic surgery procedure. The outpatient/ambulatory surgery center must be accredited or certified by the appropriate surgery center accreditation for the state. The plastic surgery nurse working in an outpatient/ambulatory surgery center maintains the plastic surgery nursing standards of practice and standards of professional performance.

Plastic Surgery Nursing: Scope and Standards of Practice 2nd Edition 13

Office-Based Surgery Centers

According to ASPS (2009) statistical data, 65% of aesthetic plastic surgery procedures and 46% of reconstructive plastic surgery procedures are performed in a plastic surgeon's office (www.asps.org). This poses risks if the office does not have a properly accredited or regulated surgery facility. Public awareness and understanding of proper accreditation and regulation is needed to provide clarity and guidance when considering plastic surgery. The plastic surgery nurse is aware of the potential confusion surrounding office-based surgery and can be instrumental in providing proper education about accreditation and regulation for other nurses, consumers, and communities.

The role of the plastic surgery nurse in the office-based surgery center includes the consultation, preoperative, postoperative, and follow-up stages of the plastic surgery procedure. The plastic surgery nurse demonstrates the appropriate skills, knowledge, competencies, and abilities to provide proper nursing care for the plastic surgery healthcare consumer. In addition to nursing responsibilities, the office-based plastic surgery nurse may have administrative responsibilities such as staffing, billing, insurance filing, verification and predetermination, as well as budgetary duties including purchasing of medical supplies and equipment.

Assessment, education, planning, and intervention are part of the plastic surgery nurse's role during each stage of a plastic surgery procedure. The plastic surgery nurse helps to improve the quality of care by maintaining standards, including the Standards of Plastic Surgery Nursing, measuring performance, and providing education within the specific office-based surgery center.

Private Practice Settings

The plastic surgery nurse working in a private practice may have responsibilities that include assessing the individual healthcare consumer's needs, developing educational material, assisting physicians or advanced practice plastic surgery nurses, and conducting staff education and in-service and healthcare consumer education. The plastic surgery nurse assesses educational needs and then provides educational material and instruction on the plastic surgery procedure. In addition, there may be management responsibilities such as billing, surgery scheduling, and insurance filing and verification, as well as budgetary duties regarding annual budgets and purchase of medical supplies and equipment.

The plastic surgery nurse also provides preoperative and postoperative counseling regarding technical aspects of the surgical procedure, documented health assessment, pertinent mutual goal planning, and psychosocial assessment and

Appendix A. Plastic Surgery Nursing: Scope and Standards of Practice (2013)

The content in this appendix is not current and is of historical significance only.

support. Other responsibilities may include sedation, postanesthesia recovery, and assisting with the procedure.

The plastic surgery nurse may provide consumer education about selecting an appropriate plastic surgery facility and provider that will meet the consumer's needs and provide the best outcomes. The plastic surgery nurse in private practice provides follow-up communication and evaluation to ensure quality of care, health maintenance, and proper documentation. The plastic surgery nurse in private practice maintains the plastic surgery nursing standards of practice and standards of professional performance.

Private practice has increasingly become an area for the aesthetic nurse specialty to practice, in collaboration with the physician. In many instances, this aesthetic nurse performs many, if not all, of the nonsurgical aesthetic enhancement procedures within the practice. In this role, the aesthetic nurse will function as counselor, provider, educator, and communicator. The aesthetic nurse maintains the plastic surgery nursing standards of practice and standards of professional and competent performance, as well as high ethical standards.

Medical Spas

New trends and increasing demands for aesthetic procedures have prompted the emergence of *medical spas*; this is a combination of a medical office and a day spa that operates under the supervision of a medical doctor. Medical spas tend to have a more clinical atmosphere than day spas, and can offer a wide range of services and treatments, including hair removal and reduction, injectables (such as botulinum toxin Type A and fillers), chemical peels, microdermabrasion, minor laser treatments, and/or sclerotherapy.

The plastic surgery nurse in the role of aesthetic nurse in these settings incorporates reputable educational preparation, such as workshops, conferences, and industry training, in learning new technologies and products relating to the procedures directly provided. The aesthetic nurse practices for a period of time directly with the supervising physician before practicing independently and is accountable for her or his practice.

Before practicing independently, the aesthetic nurse must gain the skills to assist in the care of the healthcare consumer who desires medical spa treatments and must have specialized advanced training in aesthetic nursing, including facial anatomy, assessment, products, procedures, and technology. The aesthetic nurse must maintain an active, collaborative relationship with the medical doctor of the spa. The aesthetic nurse may utilize protocols that are developed collaboratively with the medical doctor to guide practice. The aesthetic nurse should practice documentation of procedures and postprocedure follow-up. The collaborating physician should perform and document periodic supervision of the nurse's performance, to assure competency. The aesthetic nurse should be responsible for utilizing the best available evidence to guide treatment choices, should provide potential consumers with truthful information, and should not have any conflicts of interest.

Ethics and Advocacy in Plastic Surgery Nursing

Ethics is a fundamental part of nursing. Ethical awareness, judgments, and decisions are founded on a combination of principles, theories, and moral foundations. Nursing ethics are based on care and the actions of caring, to enhance and protect healthcare consumer well-being. Plastic surgery nurses are expected to comply with and promote the ethical ideals, model, code, and principles of the nursing profession. *Code of Ethics for Nurses with Interpretive Statements* (ANA, 2001) is the framework on which plastic surgery nurses base ethical analysis and decision-making, and on which standards are based. The plastic surgery nurse is also an advocate for the healthcare consumer and provides care in a nondiscriminatory and nonjudgmental way. Patient advocacy mandates preservation of autonomy, execution of clinical judgments, and management of ethical issues.

The plastic surgery nurse maintains the plastic surgery standards of practice and standards of professional performance in each type of practice environment to help ensure the safety, quality of care, and the highest level of health maintenance or health restoration for the consumer undergoing plastic surgery. The plastic surgery nurse's attitude and performance reflect compassion and understanding of a consumer's self-respect, cultural beliefs, sovereignty, and rights to self-determination and privacy. Plastic surgery nurses implement the principles of autonomy, nonmaleficence, beneficence, and justice when interacting with consumers requiring or desiring plastic surgery interventions. Plastic surgery nurses are aware of the many ethical considerations associated with the public's perception of plastic surgery, which include misleading advertising, issues affecting the aging population, insurance reimbursement, and other matters. Public awareness of these issues is the key to proper acknowledgment of the physical and emotional health concerns and risks of plastic surgery.

Misleading Advertising

Advertisements for plastic surgery are found in print, broadcast media, and the Internet. Many plastic or cosmetic surgery advertisements do not disclose risks, recovery time, contraindications, physician credentials, type of board certification, or type of surgical facility. Plastic surgery nurses encourage consumers who are interested in plastic surgery to inquire about the physician, the surgical environment, and the procedure in detail, in order to make an informed decision. Although the American Board of Plastic Surgery (www.abps .org) recognizes the role of legitimate advertising in the changing medical scene, it does not approve of plastic surgery advertising that is false or misleading and minimizes the magnitude and possible risks of surgery, or which solicits healthcare consumers for operations that they might not otherwise consider. Public awareness of plastic surgery advertising, in general, is a focus of plastic surgery nursing education in community campaigns.

The Aging Population

The quest for a more youthful appearance to complement longevity is spreading among the aging population in our society. Aging adults are considered vulnerable because of age-related physical and cognitive changes that make them more susceptible to health risks during and after surgery. According to the ASPS statistical chart for age distribution (2009), consumers aged 55 and older underwent 3.1 million total cosmetic procedures, of which 344,000 were surgical and 2.8 million were minimally invasive (www.asps.org). Cosmetic minimally invasive procedures, in general, increased 99% from 2000 to 2009. Plastic surgery nurses must be aware of the specialized needs of the aging population, as well as the ethical considerations associated with their aesthetic surgery requests.

Insurance Reimbursements

Reimbursement for plastic surgery procedures is best facilitated by educating insurance providers as to the differences between cosmetic and reconstructive surgery. Cosmetic surgery seeks to improve the patient's features on a purely aesthetic level, in the absence of any actual deformity or trauma. For this reason, insurance companies normally do not cover cosmetic surgery. In contrast, the purpose of reconstructive surgery is to correct any physical feature that is grossly deformed or abnormal by accepted standards—either as the result of a birth defect, illness, or trauma. Often, reconstructive surgery not only addresses the deformed appearance, but also seeks to correct or improve some deficiency or abnormality in function as well. A plastic surgery nurse in a plastic surgery practice environment is in a unique position to act as a consumer advocate or a change agent to help secure insurance reimbursements for those undergoing such reconstructive procedures.

Summary of the Scope of Plastic Surgery Nursing Practice

Plastic surgery nursing specializes in the protection, maintenance, safety, and optimization of health and human bodily restoration and repair before, during, and after plastic surgery cosmetic, reconstructive, and nonsurgical aesthetic procedures, regardless of the practice environment. The plastic surgery nurse collaborates, consults, and serves as a liaison and advocate for individuals, families, communities, and populations. With the dynamic and ever-changing healthcare practice environment, the plastic surgery nurse is constantly seeking to utilize the best available evidence to guide practice and promote optimal consumer outcomes for the whole person.

Standards of Plastic Surgery Nursing Practice

Standards of Practice for Plastic Surgery Nursing

Standard 1. Assessment

The plastic surgery registered nurse collects comprehensive data pertinent to the healthcare consumer's health and/or situation.

COMPETENCIES

The plastic surgery nurse:

- Collects comprehensive data, including but not limited to physical, functional, psychosocial, emotional, cognitive, sexual, cultural, age-related, environmental, spiritual/transpersonal, and economic assessments, in a systematic and ongoing process while honoring the uniqueness of the person.

- Elicits the healthcare consumer's values, preferences, expressed needs, expectations, and knowledge of the healthcare situation.

- Identifies barriers to effective communication and makes appropriate adaptations.

- Includes the healthcare consumer, family, significant others, and appropriate healthcare providers in the holistic data collection process.

- Recognizes the impact of personal attitudes, values, and beliefs.

- Prioritizes data collection.

19

- Uses appropriate evidence-based assessment techniques, analytical models and instruments, and problem-solving tools in collecting pertinent data according to the plastic surgery healthcare consumer's immediate health condition, situation, or anticipated needs.

- Synthesizes available data, information, and knowledge relevant to the situation to identify patterns and variances.

- Documents relevant data in a retrievable format.

- Applies ethical, legal, and privacy guidelines and policies to the collection, maintenance, use, and dissemination of data and information.

- Recognizes the healthcare consumer as the authority on her or his own health by honoring the consumer's care preferences.

- Assesses family dynamics and impact on healthcare consumer health and wellness.

ADDITIONAL COMPETENCIES FOR THE ADVANCED PRACTICE REGISTERED NURSE IN PLASTIC SURGERY
The advanced practice registered nurse in plastic surgery:

- Conducts in-depth and comprehensive assessments based on a synthesis of individual and family health.

- Bases assessments on advanced knowledge in the field of plastic surgery.

- Initiates and interprets diagnostic tests and procedures relevant to the current status of the plastic surgery healthcare consumer.

- Assesses the effect of interactions among individuals, family, community, and social systems on health and illness.

The content in this appendix is not current and is of historical significance only.

Appendix A. Plastic Surgery Nursing: Scope and Standards of Practice (2013)

Standard 2. Diagnosis

The plastic surgery registered nurse analyzes the assessment data to determine the diagnoses or issues.

COMPETENCIES

The plastic surgery registered nurse:

- Derives the diagnosis and issues from the assessment data obtained during interview, consultation, physical examination, diagnostic test, or diagnostic procedures.

- Identifies actual or potential risks to the healthcare consumer's health and safety, as well as barriers to health, which may include but are not limited to interpersonal, systematic, or environmental circumstances.

- Uses standardized classification systems and clinical decision support tools, when available, in identifying diagnoses.

- Bases the diagnosis on actual or potential responses to alterations in health.

- Validates the diagnoses or issues with the plastic surgery healthcare consumer, significant others, and other appropriate healthcare providers when possible.

- Documents diagnoses or issues in a manner that facilitates determination of the expected outcomes and plan.

ADDITIONAL COMPETENCIES FOR THE ADVANCED PRACTICE REGISTERED NURSE IN PLASTIC SURGERY

The advanced practice registered nurse in plastic surgery:

- Systematically compares and contrasts clinical findings of the plastic surgery patient with normal and abnormal variations and developmental events when formulating a differential diagnosis.

- Utilizes complex data and information obtained during the interview, consultation, examination, and diagnostic procedures, and initiates further appropriate diagnostic tests to complete the identification of diagnoses.

- Assists staff in building and sustaining competency in the diagnostic process.

Standard 3. Outcomes Identification

The plastic surgery registered nurse identifies expected outcomes for a plan individualized to the healthcare consumer or the situation.

COMPETENCIES

The plastic surgery registered nurse:

- Involves the healthcare consumer, family, healthcare providers, and others in formulating expected outcomes when possible and appropriate.

- Derives culturally appropriate expected outcomes from the diagnoses.

- Considers associated risks, benefits, costs, current scientific evidence, expected trajectory of the condition, and clinical expertise when formulating expected outcomes.

- Defines expected outcomes in terms of the healthcare consumer's culture, values, and ethical considerations.

- Includes a time estimate for the attainment of expected outcomes.

- Develops expected outcomes that facilitate continuity of care.

- Modifies expected outcomes based on changes in the status of the healthcare consumer or evaluation of the situation.

- Documents expected outcomes as measurable goals.

ADDITIONAL COMPETENCIES FOR THE ADVANCED PRACTICE REGISTERED NURSE IN PLASTIC SURGERY

The advanced practice registered nurse in plastic surgery:

- Identifies expected outcomes that incorporate scientific evidence and are achievable through implementation of evidence-based practices.

- Identifies expected outcomes that incorporate cost and clinical effectiveness, healthcare consumer satisfaction, and continuity and consistency among providers.

- Differentiates outcomes that require care process interventions from those that require system-level interventions.

Appendix A. Plastic Surgery Nursing: Scope and Standards of Practice (2013)

The content in this appendix is not current and is of historical significance only.

Standard 4. Planning

The plastic surgery registered nurse develops a plan that prescribes strategies and alternatives to attain expected outcomes.

COMPETENCIES

The plastic surgery registered nurse:

- Develops an individualized plan in partnership with the healthcare consumer, family, and others while considering the healthcare consumer's characteristics or situation, including but not limited to values, beliefs, spiritual and health practices, preferences, choices, developmental level, coping style, culture and environment, and available technology.

- Establishes the plan priorities with the healthcare consumer, family, and others as appropriate.

- Includes strategies in the plan that address each of the identified diagnoses or issues. These may include, but are not limited to, strategies for:

  - Promotion and restoration of health

  - Prevention of illness, injury, and disease

  - Alleviation of suffering

  - Supportive care for those who are dying

- Includes strategies for health and wholeness across the lifespan.

- Provides for continuity in the plan.

- Incorporates an implementation pathway or timeline in the plan.

- Utilizes the plan to provide direction to other members of the healthcare team.

- Explores practice settings and safe space and time for the plastic surgery registered nurse and the healthcare consumer to explore suggested, potential, and alternative options.

- Defines a plan that reflects current statutes, rules, regulations, standards, and policies.

- Modifies the plan according to ongoing assessment of the healthcare consumer's response and other outcome indicators.

- Integrates current scientific evidence, trends, and research in the planning process.

- Considers the economic impact of the plan on the plastic surgery patient, family, caregivers, and other affected parties.

- Documents the plan in a manner that uses standardized language or recognized terminology.

ADDITIONAL COMPETENCIES FOR THE ADVANCED PRACTICE REGISTERED NURSE IN PLASTIC SURGERY

The advanced practice registered nurse in plastic surgery:

- Identifies assessment and diagnostic strategies and therapeutic interventions in the plan that reflect current evidence, including data, research, literature, and expert clinical knowledge.

- Selects or designs strategies to meet the multifaceted needs of complex plastic surgery healthcare consumers.

- Includes a synthesis of the healthcare consumer's values and beliefs regarding nursing and medical therapies within the plan.

- Actively participates in the development and continuous improvement of systems that support the planning process.

- Leads the design and development of interprofessional processes to address the identified diagnosis or issue.

Standard 5. Implementation

The plastic surgery registered nurse implements the identified plan.

COMPETENCIES

The plastic surgery registered nurse:

- Partners with the person, family, significant others, and caregivers as appropriate to implement the plan in a safe, realistic, and timely manner.

- Demonstrates caring behaviors toward healthcare consumers, significant others, and groups of people receiving care.

- Utilizes technology to measure, record, and retrieve healthcare consumer data, implement the nursing process, and enhance plastic surgery nursing practice.

- Utilizes evidence-based interventions and treatments specific to the diagnosis or problem of the plastic surgery healthcare consumer.

- Provides holistic care that addresses the needs of diverse populations across the lifespan.

- Advocates for health care that is sensitive to the needs of healthcare consumers, with particular emphasis on the needs of diverse populations.

- Applies appropriate knowledge of major health problems and cultural diversity in implementing the plan of care.

- Applies available healthcare technologies to maximize access and optimize outcomes for healthcare consumers.

- Utilizes community resources and systems to implement the plan.

- Collaborates with healthcare providers from diverse backgrounds to implement and integrate the plan.

- Accommodates different styles of communication used by healthcare consumers, families, and healthcare providers.

- Integrates traditional and complementary healthcare practices as appropriate.

- Implements the plan in a timely manner in accordance with healthcare consumer safety goals.

- Promotes the healthcare consumer's capacity for the optimal level of participation and problem-solving.

- Documents implementation and any modifications, including changes or omissions, of the identified plan.

ADDITIONAL COMPETENCIES FOR THE ADVANCED PRACTICE REGISTERED NURSE IN PLASTIC SURGERY

The advanced practice registered nurse in plastic surgery:

- Facilitates utilization of systems, organizations, and community resources to implement the plan for the plastic surgery healthcare consumer.

- Supports collaboration with nursing and other colleagues to implement the plan.

- Incorporates new knowledge and strategies to initiate change in plastic surgery nursing care practices if desired outcomes are not achieved.

- Assumes responsibility for safe and efficient implementation of the plan.

- Uses advanced communication skills to promote relationships between plastic surgery nurses and healthcare consumers, to provide a context for open discussion of the healthcare consumer's experiences, and to improve healthcare consumer outcomes.

- Actively participates in the development and continuous improvement of systems that support implementation of the plan.

Standard 5A. Coordination of Care

The plastic surgery registered nurse coordinates care delivery.

COMPETENCIES

The plastic surgery registered nurse:

- Organizes the components of the plan.

- Manages a healthcare consumer's care so as to maximize independence and quality of life.

- Assists the healthcare consumer in identifying options for alternative care.

- Communicates with the healthcare consumer, family, and system during transitions in care.

- Advocates for the delivery of dignified and humane care by the interprofessional team.

- Documents the coordination of the care.

ADDITIONAL COMPETENCIES FOR THE ADVANCED
PRACTICE REGISTERED NURSE IN PLASTIC SURGERY

The advanced practice registered nurse in plastic surgery:

- Provides leadership in the coordination of interprofessional heath care for integrated delivery of plastic surgery healthcare consumer care services.

- Synthesizes data and information to prescribe necessary system and community support measures, including modifications of surroundings.

Plastic Surgery Nursing: Scope and Standards of Practice 2nd Edition   27

Standard 5B. Health Teaching and Health Promotion

The plastic surgery registered nurse employs strategies to promote health and a safe environment.

COMPETENCIES

The plastic surgery registered nurse:

- Provides health teaching that addresses such topics as healthy lifestyles, risk-reducing behaviors, developmental needs, activities of daily living, and preventive self-care.

- Uses health promotion and health teaching methods appropriate to the situation and the healthcare consumer's values, beliefs, health practices, developmental level, learning needs, readiness and ability to learn, language preference, spirituality, culture, and socioeconomic status.

- Seeks opportunities for feedback and evaluation of the effectiveness of the strategies used.

- Uses information technologies to communicate health promotion and disease prevention information to the healthcare consumer in a variety of settings.

- Provides healthcare consumers with information about intended effects and potential adverse effects of proposed therapies.

ADDITIONAL COMPETENCIES FOR THE ADVANCED PRACTICE REGISTERED NURSE IN PLASTIC SURGERY

The advanced practice registered nurse in plastic surgery:

- Synthesizes empirical evidence on risk behaviors, learning theories, behavioral change theories, motivational theories, epidemiology, and other related theories and frameworks when designing health information and programs.

- Conducts personalized health teaching and counseling in accordance with comparative effectiveness research recommendations.

- Designs health information and healthcare consumer education appropriate to the healthcare consumer's developmental level, learning needs, readiness to learn, and cultural values and beliefs.

- Evaluates health information resources, such as the Internet, within the area of plastic surgery nursing practice for accuracy, readability, and comprehensibility, to help healthcare consumers access quality health information.

- Engages consumer alliances and advocacy groups, as appropriate, in health teaching and health promotion activities.

- Provides anticipatory guidance to individuals, families, groups, and communities to promote health and prevent or reduce the risk of health problems.

Plastic Surgery Nursing: Scope and Standards of Practice 2nd Edition   29

Appendix A. Plastic Surgery Nursing: Scope and Standards of Practice (2013)

Standard 5C. Consultation

The advanced practice registered nurse in plastic surgery provides consultation to influence the specified plan, enhance the abilities of others, and effect change.

COMPETENCIES FOR THE ADVANCED PRACTICE REGISTERED NURSE

The advanced practice registered nurse in plastic surgery:

- Synthesizes clinical data, theoretical frameworks, and evidence when providing consultation.

- Facilitates the effectiveness of a consultation by involving the healthcare consumer and other stakeholders in the decision-making process and negotiating role responsibilities.

- Communicates consultation recommendations.

Standard 5D. Prescriptive Authority and Treatment

The advanced practice registered nurse in plastic surgery uses prescriptive authority, procedures, referrals, treatments, and therapies in accordance with state and federal laws and regulations.

COMPETENCIES FOR THE ADVANCED PRACTICE REGISTERED NURSE

The advanced practice registered nurse in plastic surgery:

- Prescribes evidence-based treatments, therapies, and procedures considering the healthcare consumer's comprehensive healthcare needs.

- Prescribes pharmacological agents based on current knowledge of pharmacology and physiology.

- Prescribes specific pharmacological agents and/or treatments according to clinical indicators, the healthcare consumer's status and needs, and the results of diagnostic and laboratory tests.

- Evaluates therapeutic and potential adverse effects of pharmacological and nonpharmacological treatments.

- Provides healthcare consumers with information about intended effects and potential adverse effects of proposed prescriptive therapies.

- Provides information about costs and alternative treatments and procedures, as appropriate.

- Evaluates and incorporates complementary and alternative therapy into education and practice.

Appendix A. Plastic Surgery Nursing: Scope and Standards of Practice (2013)

Standard 6. Evaluation

The plastic surgery nurse evaluates progress toward attainment of outcomes.

COMPETENCIES

The plastic surgery registered nurse:

- Conducts a systematic, ongoing, and criterion-based evaluation of the outcomes in relation to the structures and processes prescribed by the plan of care and the indicated timeline.

- Collaborates with the healthcare consumer and others involved in the care or situation in the evaluation process.

- Evaluates, in partnership with the healthcare consumer, the effectiveness of the planned strategies in relation to the healthcare consumer's responses and attainment of the expected outcomes.

- Documents the results of the evaluation.

- Uses ongoing assessment data to revise the diagnoses, outcomes, plan of care, and implementation as needed.

- Disseminates the results to the healthcare consumer, family, and others involved, in accordance with federal and state regulations.

- Participates in assessing and assuring the responsible and appropriate use of interventions in order to minimize unwarranted or unwanted treatment and healthcare consumer suffering.

ADDITIONAL COMPETENCIES FOR THE ADVANCED PRACTICE REGISTERED NURSE IN PLASTIC SURGERY

The advanced practice registered nurse in plastic surgery:

- Evaluates the accuracy of the diagnosis and effectiveness of the interventions and other variables in relation to the healthcare consumer's attainment of expected outcomes.

- Adapts the plan of care for the trajectory of treatment according to the evaluation of response.

- Synthesizes the results of the evaluation to determine the effect of the plan on healthcare consumers, families, groups, communities, and institutions.
- Uses the results of the evaluation to make or recommend process or structural changes, including policy, procedure, or protocol revision, as appropriate.

Standards of Professional Performance for Plastic Surgery Nursing

Standard 7. Ethics

The plastic surgery registered nurse practices ethically.

COMPETENCIES

The plastic surgery registered nurse:

- Uses *Code of Ethics for Nurses with Interpretive Statements* (ANA, 2001) to guide practice.

- Delivers care in a manner that preserves and protects healthcare consumer autonomy, dignity, rights, values, and beliefs.

- Recognizes the centrality of the healthcare consumer and family as core members of the healthcare team.

- Upholds healthcare consumer confidentiality within legal and regulatory parameters.

- Assists healthcare consumers in self-determination and informed decision-making.

- Maintains a therapeutic and professional healthcare consumer–nurse relationship within appropriate professional role boundaries.

- Contributes to resolving ethical issues involving healthcare consumers, colleagues, community groups, systems, and other stakeholders.

- Takes appropriate action regarding instances of illegal, unethical, or inappropriate behavior that could endanger or jeopardize the best interests of the healthcare consumer or situation.

- Speaks up as appropriate to question healthcare practice, when necessary for safety and quality improvement.

- Advocates for equitable healthcare consumer care.

Appendix A. Plastic Surgery Nursing: Scope and Standards of Practice (2013)

ADDITIONAL COMPETENCIES FOR THE ADVANCED PRACTICE REGISTERED NURSE IN PLASTIC SURGERY

The advanced practice registered nurse in plastic surgery:

- Provides information on the risks, benefits, and outcomes of the healthcare consumer regimens to allow informed decision-making by the healthcare consumer, including informed consent and informed refusal.

- Participates in interprofessional teams that address ethical risks, benefits, and outcomes.

Plastic Surgery Nursing: Scope and Standards of Practice 2nd Edition   35

Appendix A. Plastic Surgery Nursing: Scope and Standards of Practice (2013)

The content in this appendix is not current and is of historical significance only.

Standard 8. Education

The plastic surgery registered nurse attains knowledge and competence that reflect current plastic surgery nursing practice.

COMPETENCIES

The plastic surgery registered nurse:

- Participates in ongoing educational activities related to appropriate knowledge bases and professional issues.

- Demonstrates a commitment to lifelong learning through self-reflection and inquiry to address learning and personal growth needs.

- Seeks experiences that reflect current plastic surgery nursing practice, to maintain knowledge, skills, abilities, and judgment in clinical practice or role performance.

- Acquires knowledge and skills appropriate to the role, population, specialty, setting, or situation.

- Seeks formal and independent learning experiences to develop and maintain clinical and professional skills and knowledge.

- Identifies learning needs based on nursing knowledge, the various roles the plastic surgery registered nurse may assume, and the changing needs of the population.

- Participates in formal or informal consultations to address issues in plastic surgery nursing practice as an application of education and a knowledge base.

- Shares educational findings, experiences, and ideas with peers.

- Contributes to a work environment conducive to the education of healthcare professionals.

- Maintains professional records that provide evidence of competence and lifelong learning.

ADDITIONAL COMPETENCIES FOR THE ADVANCED PRACTICE REGISTERED NURSE IN PLASTIC SURGERY

The advanced practice registered nurse in plastic surgery:

- Uses current healthcare research findings and other evidence to expand clinical knowledge, skills, abilities, and judgment to enhance role performance, and to increase knowledge of professional issues.

Plastic Surgery Nursing: Scope and Standards of Practice 2nd Edition   37

Appendix A. Plastic Surgery Nursing: Scope and Standards of Practice (2013)

Standard 9. Evidence-Based Practice and Research

The plastic surgery registered nurse integrates evidence and research findings into practice.

COMPETENCIES

The plastic surgery registered nurse:

- Utilizes current evidence-based nursing knowledge, including research findings, to guide practice.

- Incorporates evidence when initiating changes in plastic surgery nursing practice.

- Participates, as appropriate to education level and position, in the formulation of evidence-based practice through research.

- Shares personal and third-party research findings with colleagues and peers.

ADDITIONAL COMPETENCIES FOR THE ADVANCED PRACTICE REGISTERED NURSE IN PLASTIC SURGERY

The advanced practice registered nurse in plastic surgery:

- Contributes to plastic surgery nursing knowledge by conducting or synthesizing research and other evidence that discovers, examines, and evaluates current practice, knowledge, theories, criteria, and creative approaches to improve healthcare outcomes.

- Promotes a climate of research and clinical inquiry.

- Disseminates research findings through activities such as presentations, publications, consultation, and journal clubs.

Appendix A. Plastic Surgery Nursing: Scope and Standards of Practice (2013)

Standard 10. Quality of Practice

The plastic surgery registered nurse contributes to quality nursing practice.

COMPETENCIES

The plastic surgery registered nurse:

- Demonstrates quality by documenting the application of the nursing process in a responsible, accountable, and ethical manner,

- Uses creativity and innovation to enhance plastic surgery nursing care.

- Participates in quality improvement activities, such as but not limited to:

  - Identifying aspects of practice important for quality monitoring

  - Using indicators to monitor quality, safety, and effectiveness of plastic surgery nursing practice

  - Collecting data to monitor quality and effectiveness of plastic surgery nursing practice

  - Analyzing quality data to identify opportunities for improving plastic surgery nursing practice

  - Formulating recommendations to improve plastic surgery nursing practice or outcomes

  - Implementing activities to enhance the quality of plastic surgery nursing practice

  - Developing, implementing, and/or evaluating policies, procedures, and guidelines to improve the quality of practice

  - Participating in and/or leading interprofessional teams to evaluate clinical care or health services

  - Participating in and/or leading efforts to minimize costs and unnecessary duplication

  - Identifying problems that occur in day-to-day work routines, in order to correct process inefficiencies

  - Analyzing factors related to quality, safety, and effectiveness

- Analyzing organizational systems for barriers to quality healthcare consumer outcomes

- Implementing processes to remove or weaken barriers within organizational systems

- Obtains and maintains professional certification in plastic surgery nursing.

ADDITIONAL COMPETENCIES FOR THE ADVANCED PRACTICE REGISTERED NURSE IN PLASTIC SURGERY

The advanced practice registered nurse in plastic surgery:

- Provides leadership in design and implementation of quality improvements.

- Designs innovations to effect change in practice and improve health outcomes.

- Evaluates the practice environment and quality of nursing care rendered in relation to existing evidence.

- Identifies opportunities for the generation and use of research and evidence.

- Obtains and maintains professional certification.

- Uses the results of quality improvement to initiate changes in plastic surgery nursing practice and the healthcare delivery system.

Standard 11. Communication

The plastic surgery registered nurse communicates effectively in a variety of formats in all areas of practice.

COMPETENCIES

The plastic surgery registered nurse:

- Assesses communication format preferences of healthcare consumers, families, and colleagues.

- Assesses her or his own communication skills in encounters with healthcare consumers, families, and colleagues.

- Seeks continuous improvement of communication and conflict resolution skills.

- Conveys information to healthcare consumers, families, the interprofessional team, and others in communication formats that promote accuracy.

- Questions the rationale supporting care processes and decisions when they do not appear to be in the best interest of the plastic surgery healthcare consumer.

- Discloses observations or concerns related to hazards and errors in care or the practice environment to the appropriate level.

- Maintains communication with other providers to minimize risks associated with transfers and transition in care delivery.

- Contributes her or his own professional perspective in discussions with the interprofessional team.

Plastic Surgery Nursing: Scope and Standards of Practice 2nd Edition   41

Standard 12. Leadership

The plastic surgery nurse demonstrates leadership in the professional practice setting and in the profession.

COMPETENCIES
The plastic surgery registered nurse:

- Oversees the nursing care given by others while retaining accountability for the quality of care given to the healthcare consumer.

- Abides by the vision, the associated goals, and the plan to implement and measure progress of an individual healthcare consumer or progress within the context of the healthcare organization.

- Demonstrates a commitment to continuous, lifelong learning and education for self and others.

- Mentors colleagues for advancement of plastic surgery nursing practice, the profession, and quality health care.

- Treats colleagues with respect, trust, and dignity.

- Develops communication and conflict resolution skills.

- Participates in professional organizations, including the American Society of Plastic Surgical Nurses.

- Communicates effectively with the healthcare consumer and colleagues.

- Seeks ways to advance plastic surgery nursing autonomy and accountability.

- Participates in efforts to influence healthcare policy involving healthcare consumers and plastic surgery nursing.

ADDITIONAL COMPETENCIES FOR THE ADVANCED PRACTICE REGISTERED NURSE IN PLASTIC SURGERY
The advanced practice registered nurse in plastic surgery:

- Influences decision-making bodies to improve the professional practice environment and healthcare consumer outcomes.

- Provides direction to enhance the effectiveness of the interprofessional team.

The content in this appendix is not current and is of historical significance only.

Appendix A. Plastic Surgery Nursing: Scope and Standards of Practice (2013)

- Promotes advanced practice in plastic surgery nursing and role development by interpreting its role for the healthcare consumer, families, and others.

- Models expert practice to interprofessional team members and healthcare consumers.

- Mentors colleagues in the acquisition of clinical knowledge, skills, abilities, and judgment.

Plastic Surgery Nursing: Scope and Standards of Practice 2nd Edition   43

Standard 13. Collaboration

The plastic surgery registered nurse collaborates with the healthcare consumer, family, and others in the conduct of plastic surgery nursing practice.

COMPETENCIES
The plastic surgery registered nurse:

- Partners with others to effect change and produce positive outcomes through sharing of knowledge of the healthcare consumer and/or situation.

- Communicates with the healthcare consumer, family, and healthcare providers regarding healthcare consumer care and the plastic surgery registered nurse's role in the provision of that care.

- Promotes conflict management and engagement.

- Participates in building consensus or resolving conflict in the context of patient care.

- Applies group process and negotiation techniques with healthcare consumers and colleagues.

- Adheres to standards and applicable codes of conduct that govern behavior among peers and colleagues, so as to create a work environment that promotes cooperation, respect, and trust.

- Cooperates in creating a documented plan focused on outcomes and decisions related to care and delivery of services that indicates communication with healthcare consumers, families, and others.

- Engages in teamwork and team-building processes.

ADDITIONAL COMPETENCIES FOR THE ADVANCED PRACTICE REGISTERED NURSE IN PLASTIC SURGERY
The advanced practice registered nurse in plastic surgery:

- Partners with other disciplines to enhance healthcare consumer outcomes through interprofessional activities, such as education, consultation, management, technological development, or research opportunities.

- Invites the contribution of the healthcare consumer, family, and team members in order to achieve optimal outcomes.

- Leads in establishing, improving, and sustaining collaborative relationships to achieve safe, quality healthcare consumer care.

- Documents plan-of-care communications, rationales for plan-of-care changes, and collaborative discussions to improve healthcare consumer outcomes.

Standard 14. Professional Practice Evaluation

The plastic surgery registered nurse evaluates her or his own nursing practice in relation to professional practice standards and guidelines, relevant statutes, rules, and regulations.

COMPETENCIES

The plastic surgery registered nurse:

- Provides age-appropriate and developmentally appropriate care in a culturally and ethnically sensitive manner.

- Engages in self-evaluation of practice on a regular basis, identifying areas of strength as well as areas in which professional growth would be beneficial.

- Obtains informal feedback regarding her or his own practice from healthcare consumers, peers, professional colleagues, and others.

- Participates in peer review as appropriate.

- Takes action to achieve goals identified during the evaluation process.

- Provides the evidence for practice decisions and actions as part of the informal and formal evaluation processes.

- Interacts with peers and colleagues to enhance her or his own professional nursing practice or role performance.

- Provides peers with formal or informal constructive feedback regarding their practice and role performance.

ADDITIONAL COMPETENCIES FOR THE ADVANCED PRACTICE REGISTERED NURSE IN PLASTIC SURGERY

The advanced practice registered nurse in plastic surgery:

- Engages in a formal process of seeking feedback regarding her or his own practice from healthcare consumers, peers, professional colleagues, and others.

Appendix A. Plastic Surgery Nursing: Scope and Standards of Practice (2013)

The content in this appendix is not current and is of historical significance only.

Standard 15. Resource Utilization

The plastic surgery registered nurse utilizes appropriate resources to plan and provide nursing services that are safe, effective, and financially responsible.

COMPETENCIES

The plastic surgery registered nurse:

- Assesses individual healthcare consumer care needs and resources available to achieve desired outcomes.

- Identifies healthcare consumer care needs, potential for harm, complexity of the task, and desired outcome when considering resource allocation.

- Delegates elements of care to appropriate healthcare workers in accordance with any applicable legal or policy parameters or principles.

- Identifies the evidence when evaluating resources.

- Advocates for resources, including technology, that enhance plastic surgery nursing practice.

- Modifies practice when necessary to promote positive interaction between healthcare consumers, care providers, and technology.

- Assists the healthcare consumer and family in identifying and securing appropriate services to address needs across the healthcare continuum.

- Assists the healthcare consumer and family in factoring costs, risks, and benefits in decisions about treatment and care.

ADDITIONAL COMPETENCIES FOR THE ADVANCED PRACTICE REGISTERED NURSE IN PLASTIC SURGERY

The advanced practice registered nurse in plastic surgery:

- Utilizes organizational and community resources to formulate interprofessional plans of care.

- Formulates innovative solutions for healthcare consumer care problems that utilize resources effectively and maintain quality.

- Designs evaluation strategies to demonstrate cost effectiveness, cost benefit, and efficiency factors associated with plastic surgery nursing practice.

Plastic Surgery Nursing: Scope and Standards of Practice 2nd Edition   47

Standard 16. Environmental Health

The plastic surgery registered nurse practices in an environmentally safe and healthy manner.

COMPETENCIES

The plastic surgery registered nurse:

- Attains knowledge of environmental health concepts, such as implementation of environmental health strategies.

- Promotes a practice environment that reduces environmental health risks for workers and healthcare consumers.

- Assesses the practice environment for factors that threaten health, such as sound, odor, noise, and light.

- Advocates for the judicious and appropriate use of products in health care.

- Communicates environmental health risks and exposure reduction strategies to healthcare consumers, families, colleagues, and communities.

- Utilizes scientific evidence to determine if a product or treatment is an environmental threat.

- Participates in strategies to promote healthy communities.

ADDITIONAL COMPETENCIES FOR THE ADVANCED PRACTICE REGISTERED NURSE IN PLASTIC SURGERY

The advanced practice registered nurse in plastic surgery:

- Creates partnerships that promote sustainable environmental health policies and conditions.

- Analyzes the impact of social, political, and economic influences on the environment and human health exposures.

- Critically evaluates the manner in which environmental health issues are presented by the popular media.

- Advocates for implementation of environmental principles for plastic surgery nursing practice.

- Supports nurses in advocating for and implementing environmental principles in plastic surgery nursing practice.

The content in this appendix is not current and is of historical significance only.

Glossary

Competency. An expected and measurable level of nursing performance that integrates knowledge, skills, abilities, and judgment, based on established scientific knowledge and expectations for nursing practice.

Environment. The surrounding context, milieu, conditions, or atmosphere in which a plastic surgery nurse practices.

Evidence-based practice. A scholarly and systematic problem-solving paradigm that results in the delivery of high-quality health care.

Healthcare team. A set of individuals with special expertise who provide healthcare services or assistance to patients. They may include nurses, physicians, psychologists, social workers, nutritionists/dieticians, and various therapists. Healthcare providers also may include service organizations and vendors. A team is comprised of a number of persons associated together in work or activity.

Holism (holistic). A view of everything in terms of patterns and processes that combine to form a whole, instead of seeing things as fragments, pieces, or parts. Holistic nursing embraces nursing practice, which has healing the whole person as its goal. Holism involves understanding the individual as an integrated whole interacting with and being acted upon by both internal and external environments.

Interprofessional. Reliant on the overlapping knowledge, skills, and abilities of each professional team member. Interprofessionalism can drive synergistic effects by which outcomes are enhanced and become more comprehensive than a simple aggregation of the individual efforts of the team members.

49

Plastic surgery nursing. An area of nursing that specializes in the protection, maintenance, safety, and optimization of human bodily repair, restoration, and health before, during, and after plastic surgery procedures. This is accomplished through the nursing process, nursing diagnosis, and treatment of human response.

Role. A function; specifically, the characteristic and expected social behavior of an individual in relationship to a group.

Standards. Authoritative statements defined and promoted by a profession by which the quality of practice, service, or education can be evaluated.

Appendix A. Plastic Surgery Nursing: Scope and Standards of Practice (2013)

References

American Board of Medical Specialties (ABMS). (2000). *Member boards and associate members.* Available at http://www.abms.org/member.asp

American Board of Plastic Surgery. (2011). *About ABPS.* Available at http://www.abplsurg.org/about_abps.html#Description%20of%20Plastic%20Surgery

American Nurses Association (ANA). (2001). *Code of Ethics for Nurses with interpretive statements.* Washington, DC: ANA.

American Nurses Association (ANA). (2010a). *Nursing: Scope and standards of practice, 2nd ed.* Silver Spring, MD: Nursesbooks.org.

American Nurses Association (ANA). (2010b). *Nursing's social policy statement: The essence of the profession.* Silver Spring, MD: Nursesbooks.org

Association of periOperative Registered Nurses (AORN). (2011). *Standards and recommended practices.* Available at www.aorn.org

American Society of Plastic Surgeons. (2009). *Plastic surgery procedural statistics.* Available at http://www.plasticsurgery.org/News-and-Resources/Statistics.html

American Society of Plastic Surgical Nurses (ASPSN). (2010). *About ASPSN.* Available at http://www.aspsn.org/ABOUT/objectives.html

51

Index

P

pain management 11–12

patients. *See* clients

pediatric clients 8

piercing, body 9–10

plan of care 7, 45, 47, 55

plastic and aesthetic nurses 1

    advanced practice roles 16–17

    as educators 17–19

    healthcare clients and 7–12

    practice environments for 20–21

    roles of 14–19

plastic and aesthetic nursing

    chronology table 6

    definition of 1

    development of 5–7

    educational preparation for 12.
        See also graduate-level
        prepared RN competencies

    ethics and advocacy in 23

    explications 23–30

    foundation of 1–2

    growth of 2–3

    research and evidence-based
        practice 21–23

    scope of 31

    standards of practice for 17, 18,
        33–47

    standards of professional
        performance for 48–67

Plastic Surgical Nursing 5

Plastic Surgical Nursing Certification
    Board (PSNCB) 12

practice environment 20, 56, 62, 67.
    See also evidence-based practice
    (EBP)

primary care provider 44

private practice 20

procedures, most commonly
    requested 2–3

psychiatric diseases 22

Q

quality of life 21, 30–31, 44

R

reconstructive surgery 30–31

regulations and laws 43, 44

relationships, therapeutic 41, 42, 48

research 28, 59–60, 62

responsibilities

    administrative 20

    fiscal 65

risk factors 45–46, 67

RNs. *See also* APRNs, role of; nurse
    practitioners (NPs)

    aesthetic 2, 19, 22

    self-care 27, 48

    values and beliefs of 50. *See
        also* cultural values and
        diversity

    work life balance 27

S

safety of clients 2, 7, 23, 26

scope of practice 10–11, 14, 19

    decision tree 14

skin care

    clinical services 20

    education 20

    health intervention 27

social justice 29–30, 49

spas 20

standards of care 14, 18, 23

Standards of Plastic and Aesthetic
Nursing Practice

    assessment 33–35

    collaboration 54

    communication 52–53

    coordination of care 44

    culturally congruent
       practice 50–51

    diagnosis 36–37

    education 58

    environmental heath 67

    ethics 48–49

    evaluation 47

    evidence-based practice and
       research 59–60

    health teaching and health
       promotion 45–46

    implementation 42

    leadership 56–57

    outcomes identification 38–39

    planning 40–41

    professional practice
       evaluation 64

    quality of practice 61–63

    resource utilization 65–66

surgery. *See also* cosmetic surgery

    breast augmentation 2, 22

breast reduction 30

gender confirming 11, 30

liposuction 2, 30

most commonly requested 2–3

reconstructive 30–31

unrealistic expectations 22

systems and processes, development
   of 41, 62

T

tattoos 10

teams. *See* interprofessional collaboration

therapeutic relationships 41, 42, 48

transgender clients 11, 30

translators 52

U

unrealistic expectations

    aging and 8

    body image and 11

    for surgical or secondary
      results 22

U.S. Food and Drug Administration
   (FDA) 16

W

work life balance 27